Stop Vision Loss Now!

*Prevent and Heal
Cataracts, Glaucoma,
Macular Degeneration,
and Other Common
Eye Disorders*

Bruce Fife, ND

Piccadilly Books, Ltd.
Colorado Springs, CO

Every effort has been made to ensure that the information contained in this book is complete and accurate. However, neither the publisher nor the author is engaged in rendering professional advice or services to the individual reader. The ideas, procedures, and suggestions contained in this book are not intended as a substitute for consulting with your physician. All matters regarding your health require medical supervision. Neither the author nor the publisher shall be liable or responsible for any loss or damage allegedly arising from any information or suggestion in this book.

Piccadilly Books, Ltd.
P.O. Box 25203
Colorado Springs, CO 80936, USA
info@piccadillybooks.com
www.piccadillybooks.com

Library of Congress Cataloging-in-Publication Data
Fife, Bruce, 1952-
  Stop vision loss now! : prevent and heal cataracts, glaucoma, macular degeneration, and other common eye disorders / by Bruce Fife, ND.
     pages cm
  Includes bibliographical references and index.
  ISBN 978-0-941599-96-2
  1. Vision disorders--Prevention--Popular works. 2. Eye--Diseases--Prevention--Popular works. 3. Eye--Diseases--Nutritional aspects--Popular works. I. Title.
  RE51.F53 2015
  617.7'1--dc23
                              2014049177
Printed in the USA

Table of Contents

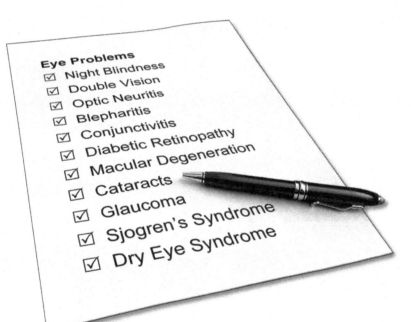

Eye Problems
- ☑ Night Blindness
- ☑ Double Vision
- ☑ Optic Neuritis
- ☑ Blepharitis
- ☑ Conjunctivitis
- ☑ Diabetic Retinopathy
- ☑ Macular Degeneration
- ☑ Cataracts
- ☑ Glaucoma
- ☑ Sjogren's Syndrome
- ☑ Dry Eye Syndrome

1

A Natural Solution
to Common Eye Problems

AN ALL-TOO-COMMON STORY

Twelve years ago, Tom McCarville owned a successful media business specializing in movie, television, and commercial photography. "One day I was in a mall and decided to do something about my un-hip eyeglass frames," says Tom. "I had to have an exam, and they did the 'poof' test—the one in which they check the pressure of your eyes by using jets of air directed at your eye. Well, they poofed and poofed and poofed. Then they asked me if I'd been tested for glaucoma recently, which I hadn't, and they recommended I go to see an ophthalmologist—which I did the next day!"

The ophthalmologist discovered that Tom's eye pressure was more than double the healthy norm, and he had permanently lost 20 percent of his peripheral, or side, vision. Tom was diagnosed with glaucoma, a degenerative eye disease that slowly destroys peripheral vision, leading to tunnel vision and eventual blindness. Nearly three million people in the United States have glaucoma, but half do not realize it because there are generally no warning signs or obvious symptoms until the disease becomes advanced.

"The disease is out of control," Tom was told. He was in shock. "I'd only gone to the doctor to get some new eyeglass frames. I had no idea that anything was wrong with my eyes." As a photographer, he relied mostly on his central vision every day, and the disease progressed so slowly over the years that he was totally unaware that he was losing his eyesight.

Glaucoma is generally considered a disease that occurs in the elderly, not in a healthy 34-year-old. There is no medical cure for glaucoma; once sight is lost, it is considered gone forever. Treatment is focused on reducing eye pressure to slow the progression of the disease. The prescription drugs Tom was given either didn't work, or, if they did work, caused terrible reactions. The pressure in his eyes remained elevated. He tried surgery to reduce the pressure, but a tear developed under his macula—the part of the retina that provides clear central vision, and that only left him with more vision problems.

"In my left eye, there are areas where I have holes in my vision. I have lots of floaters, and I know I'm developing cataracts, but if I take the time, I can see and do most everything. It's just that it takes me longer than most people." Tom had to give up his photography business. He went back to school to learn braille and other skills to help cope with everyday tasks as his eyesight worsened.

The really sad part about this story is that Tom didn't have to lose his eyesight. If he had undergone eye exams on a regular basis, his glaucoma could have been spotted early on, and steps could have been taken at that time to resolve the problem. Although Tom followed standard medical protocols, the disease continued to progress. Drugs and surgery didn't help because they do not address the underlying cause of the problem. Treating symptoms will not stop the progression of a disease, let alone reverse it.

Perhaps you know someone who has gone through or is going through a similar situation. It may not be glaucoma but some other serious eye condition that can lead to vision loss. You may even be experiencing visual difficulties yourself. The good news is that you can stop age-related vision loss, without dangerous drugs or invasive surgery. Age-related vision loss is not caused by a drug or surgery deficiency; rather, it is caused by lifestyle factors that can be easily changed. In this book, you will learn the basic underlying causes of the most common age-related eye disorders and what you can do to prevent, stop, and reverse them.

VISION LOSS CAN BE STOPPED

Of your five senses—taste, touch, sight, smell, and hearing—which is the most important to you? Which one would you most hate to lose? While all of these are important and enhance our quality of life, I think most people would agree that sight is their most cherished sense. So much of the joy we experience in life is taken in through the eyes, so the thought of losing our ability to see is horrible. Yet, every five seconds, somewhere in the world, someone succumbs to blindness. In fact, nearly 7 million people worldwide lose their sight each year. While blindness can occur due to injury or infection, most people lose their sight due to a variety of eye disorders, and the risk of vision loss and blindness increases as we age.

A survey of 1,000 adults shows that nearly half—47 percent—worry more about losing their sight than they do about losing their memory or their ability to walk or hear. Among the elderly, vision loss is the second-greatest fear, next to death.

Most eye disorders come without warning. There is no way to pre-diagnose, no way to predict who will develop age-related macular degeneration or glaucoma as they get older. Everyone is at risk, and once the disease is present, drugs, surgery, and other medical procedures are needed to slow the progression of the disease. Unfortunately, even with the latest medical treatments, these diseases may still progress to severe vision loss. There is no cure for most degenerative eye disorders, and most conventional treatments are often accompanied by potentially serious side effects. For all these reasons, prevention is the best approach, as is the case with most diseases.

However, while there may be no drugs or medical treatments that can cure these diseases, that does not mean there is no hope. There actually is an effective treatment for most common chronic eye disorders, and it does not involve drugs, surgery, or any invasive or costly medical treatment. It is based on diet. The key component of this diet is coconut oil. Coconut oil and a proper diet have been very successful in not only stopping the progression of these diseases but even reversing them. In some cases, it has done the seemingly impossible, completely eliminating the disease, as it did for me, in my own run-in with glaucoma. The success of the treatment depends on the severity of the disease, the length of time a person has suffered from the disease, and how closely the individual follows the treatment program.

THE MAGIC OF COCONUT OIL

This dietary program was the direct result of a presentation I gave to the Ocular Nutrition Society at the American Academy of Optometry annual meeting in Denver, Colorado, USA in 2014.

In May of that year, I was contacted by a representative of the Ocular Nutrition Society, an organization of eye care professionals interested in nutritional approaches to treating visual disorders. I was asked to give a lecture at their annual symposium on the benefits of coconut oil and how it may be related to improved eye health.

I was invited because I am the founder and director of the Coconut Research Center, a not-for-profit organization dedicated to teaching medical professionals and the general public about the nutritional and medicinal benefits of coconut oil and related products. I've also written a dozen books on the use of these products for the treatment of various health issues. One of my books, *Stop Alzheimer's Now!*, describes how to use coconut oil to prevent and even reverse Alzheimer's and other neurodegenerative diseases. The science behind the use of coconut oil for brain health is well established, and the success stories are truly amazing. Alzheimer's disease is being reversed, something medical science has always believed to be impossible; a simple coconut oil-based dietary program is now doing what no drug or therapy has been able to accomplish.

In 2014, however, there was still little research demonstrating a direct connection between eye heath and the use of coconut oil. The Ocular Nutrition Society representative acknowledged that fact but indicated an interest because of the remarkable effects coconut oil was having in the treatment of brain disorders such as Alzheimer's and epilepsy. The eyes are extensions of the brain, so any treatment that improves brain health is potentially of great interest to eye specialists.

I accepted the invitation and began thinking of all the ways coconut oil might help with visual problems. A characteristic of the oil is that it improves the absorption of the nutrients in the foods it is added to. Studies have shown that simply adding coconut oil to foods greatly increases the absorption of vitamins, minerals, and antioxidants, including vitamin A and lutein, two nutrients critically important to good eye health. Coconut oil, therefore, can be of potential use in protecting against eye problems associated with nutrient deficiencies.

Diabetics are at high risk of developing visual problems due to poor circulation and nerve damage associated with the disease. The disease causes nerves to degenerate throughout the body, leading to peripheral neuropathy (loss of feeling in the feet and legs), retinopathy (loss of eyesight), nephropathy (loss of kidney function), and other problems. Coconut oil is known to improve circulation and revitalize nerve function in diabetics, often reversing these conditions. Diabetics are also at high risk of developing cataracts and glaucoma. Coconut oil is effective in helping to control blood sugar and insulin levels, thus reducing the risk of these conditions in diabetics. Considering all these factors, I was sure coconut oil could be of great help in preventing and perhaps even reversing eye problems associated with diabetes.

I was also aware that diet has a strong impact on various eye conditions. Cataract is caused by free-radical damage to the lens of the eye. Free radicals, chronic inflammation, and insulin resistance can all contribute to the development of glaucoma, macular degeneration, Sjogren's syndrome, and other eye diseases. Removing certain foods and food additives that promote these conditions and replacing them with more healthful diet choices can greatly improve eye health. Major dietary changes can play a significant role in eye health, and a very beneficial one is switching from using processed vegetable oils to coconut oil. While processed vegetable oils promote free-radical degeneration associated with so many eye problems, coconut oil can act as a protective antioxidant, preventing the damage caused by free radicals. It also possesses anti-inflammatory properties to calm runaway inflammation and has shown to reverse insulin resistance. A coconut oil-based diet has the potential to help protect against a variety of eye problems.

The most amazing thing about coconut oil, however, is its ability to restore nerve and brain function. Coconut oil has proven remarkably successful in the treatment of epilepsy, Alzheimer's, Parkinson's, and other neurological disorders. Since the 1970s, it has been used as part of a dietary treatment for epilepsy. More recently it has gained a reputation as an effective treatment for Alzheimer's. Coconut oil has proven effective not only for stopping the progression of the disease but also reversing it, something no drug or medical treatment has ever come close to doing. The reason it works so well is because when ingested, coconut oil initiates a series of reactions in the body that triggers the activation of special proteins in the brain called brain derived neurotrophic factors (BDNFs). When activated, BDNFs stimulate nerve cell growth, repair, and regeneration. As mentioned, the eyes are extensions of the brain, and the retina itself is part of the optic nerve. BDNFs repair and regenerate nerves, including the optic nerve and retina. I realized that coconut oil can not only help prevent many common eye disorders but can also initiate processes that might actually restore vision.

Wow! For years we've been led to believe that once you start to lose your eyesight, it's gone for good. The same was said about the brain, that brain cells don't regenerate and that the brain cells we are born with are all we will ever have. This false notion is not true either, for brain cells do regenerate. In fact, the brain contains stem cells that, when activated, can transform into any type of cell. The process of brain cell regeneration is called neurogenesis. Like other nerve cells in the brain, the retina can be healed, potentially restoring eyesight.

MY AHA MOMENT

While I was processing this information in my mind, I realized I was a perfect example of the power of coconut oil curing eye disease, something I had failed to realize before.

Years earlier, my eyesight had been getting noticeably worse over a period of time. It had been years since my last eye exam, and I decided it was about time to see the doctor for a stronger prescription for my glasses.

When I saw the optometrist, he ran me through the standard eye exam, including the routine test for glaucoma. He tested both of my eyes, then stopped and said, "I want to check your eyes again." After the second evaluation, he looked at me with concern on his face. "I believe you might have glaucoma," he said. I was stunned, knowing that this serious condition could lead to blindness. "You need to see a specialist to confirm this," he said. I made an appointment to see an ophthalmologist.

The second doctor's diagnosis wasn't comforting, as he informed me that I was in the beginning stages of glaucoma. Since the condition wasn't critical yet, I had some time to think about how I was going to handle the problem.

At that same time, I was just beginning to learn about the benefits of coconut oil and the hazards of eating processed vegetable oils. I gradually changed my diet, eliminated vegetable oils, margarine, shortening, and any foods containing hydrogenated vegetable oil, and substituted them with coconut oil. I also started exercising regularly on a rebounder (mini-trampoline), for I had heard that it could help strengthen the eyes and improve nearsightedness, which I'd had since I was in the third grade. I got a new pair of eyeglasses with a stronger prescription, but I delayed doing anything about the glaucoma, hoping that my new diet and exercise routine might have a positive effect on my eyesight.

Over the next two years, I noticed that my eyesight was slowly changing. My vision was becoming distorted, and I was having difficulty seeing as clearly as I had before. I needed to get another eye examine and probably a stronger, prescription. I also wanted to know if my glaucoma had gotten any worse, especially since my eyesight seemed to be going downhill. A friend referred me to a different optometrist, and I made an appointment to see him. I decided not to tell the new doctor about my prior experience, as I was curious to see what he would find without being influenced by my previous diagnosis. We went through the entire exam, including the glaucoma test, and he did not seem the least bit alarmed. Since he didn't say anything about me testing positive for glaucoma, I asked, "How was my glaucoma test?"

Much to my delight, he said, "Your eyes are healthy, with no sign of glaucoma." He then added, "Interestingly, most people's eyesight gets worse as they age, but yours seems to have improved since you got your last prescription."

Remarkable! The reason my eyesight was a little distorted was because my sight had improved, and the glasses I was wearing were now too strong for my eyes. I did get a new prescription, but it was a weaker one, and I was overjoyed.

That happened about eighteen years ago, and since then, I've been back to the optometrist from time to time for checkups. Each time, he runs the glaucoma test, and each time, I pass with flying colors.

Initially, I attributed my improved eye heath to my dietary changes and regular exercise. I am certain these healthy measures did help, but as I've learned more about the remarkable effects of coconut oil, I now realize that it was probably the coconut oil that contributed the most, especially in regard to glaucoma.

Over the years, my nearsightedness has not improved any further but it has remained stable; the glasses I wear now are the same prescription I was given 18 years ago. Typically, eyesight declines with age, but at 62, my eyes are essentially the same as they were at 44. Thank you, coconut oil!

THERE IS HOPE

While there are no medical cures for most common eye disorders, there is a treatment that can help. This treatment does not depend on drugs, surgery, or any medical intervention; it is based on diet. The coconut oil-based dietary program described in this book has the potential to help prevent and reverse many common visual problems, including:

Cataracts
Glaucoma
Macular degeneration
Diabetic retinopathy
Dry eye syndrome
Sjogren's syndrome
Optic neuritis
Irritated eyes
Conjunctivitis (pink eye)
Stroke
Eye disorders related to neurodegenerative disease (Alzheimer's, Parkinson's, MS)

This is certainly not a complete list of conditions that can be helped with the use of coconut oil and a proper diet. Potentially any condition involving chronic inflammation, free-radical damage, or degeneration to the retina or optic nerve can benefit.

This book offers hope to those people who are already affected by these conditions as well as to those who are at risk of developing one or more of them in the near future. I will explain how you can tell if you are at risk before obvious symptoms arise. Most chronic eye disorders strike without warning and none of us can tell who will develop a visual handicap as we age. Everybody is at risk, and once the disease is diagnosed, treatment can be a lifelong process. In this book, you will learn the basic underlying causes for the most common degenerative eye disorders, what to look for even before the eye doctor can detect any clear signs or symptoms, and what you can do to prevent, stop, and even reverse them.

Because the suggestions in this book focus on inexpensive, natural procedures, some people may be skeptical. Can a natural approach be better than drugs that have been extensively tested and studied? Critics may question the use of coconut oil for the treatment of various visual problems, stating that there are not enough good-quality studies to prove, beyond doubt, that it is safe or effective. I admit that there are not a lot of studies specifically intended to evaluate the effects of coconut oil on visual problems; however, a multitude of studies have shown coconut oil to be completely nontoxic and safe, even in large doses, proving safety concerns invalid. But is it effective? A number of studies have shown that coconut oil provides numerous health benefits that can support good eye health and protect eyes from degenerative damage that might otherwise lead to poor eyesight and blindness. Evidence shows a distinct connection between coconut oil and the activation of BDNFs, which are known to stimulate retina growth and repair. In spite of what some so-called experts claim, we actually do have enough scientific evidence to show that coconut oil has the potential to help protect and restore vision.

Since coconut oil is completely harmless, there is no reason not to give it a try. The worst it can do is nothing; meaning you might not see the improvement you wanted, but it won't cause any harm. The best it could do for you is restore your vision, a remarkable result that is usually not possible, even with drugs and surgery. Even a partial improvement is better than no improvement at all. If it only stops the progression of your vision loss, you still benefit. Give it a try! You have nothing to lose.

Keep in mind, following the suggestions in this book does not exclude you from following your doctor's advice or perusing standard medical treatment. It may be advisable to do both, to take a more holistic approach for the sake of your eyes. Ultimately, the choice is yours, but you will never know if these methods will help you unless you give them a try.

2

The Human Eye

ANATOMY OF THE EYE

The eyes are part of the brain; during fetal development, a small part of the brain pouches out to become the eyeball and optic nerve. In essence, when you look into a person's eyes, you are seeing part of their brain.

The eye is composed of many different parts, all of which work together to enable us to see. If any one of these parts doesn't work properly or communicate well with the brain, vision can be impaired. To understand the different forms of vision loss, it's helpful to understand the anatomy of the eye, the functions of the various parts, and the associated terminology.

The eyes are extensions of the brain. The optic nerve stretches from the retina to an area of the brain called the lateral geniculate nucleus. The visual signals are then relayed to the visual cortex for interpretation.

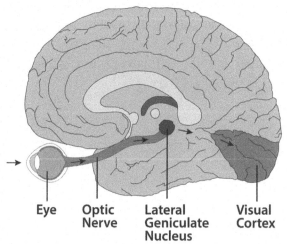

| Eye | Optic Nerve | Lateral Geniculate Nucleus | Visual Cortex |

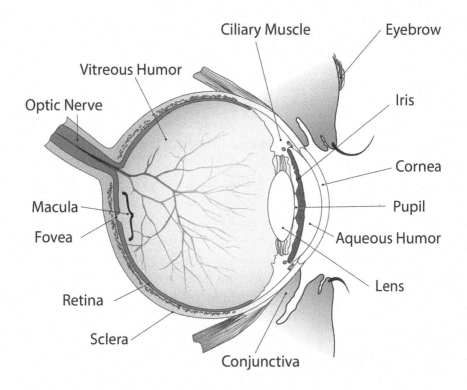

Ciliary Muscle Eyebrow

Vitreous Humor

Optic Nerve Iris

Macula Cornea

Fovea Pupil

Aqueous Humor

Retina Lens

Sclera

Conjunctiva

The eyeball is similar in size and shape to a ping-pong ball. When you look at a person's eye, you only see a small part of it. The majority of the ball-shaped eye is set inside the eye socket of the skull, hidden from view. The white part of the eye, some of which is visible, is called the **sclera**. The sclera is a tough outer membrane that encapsulates the entire eyeball, except at the very front. At the front and center of the eye, the sclera transforms into a transparent membrane called the **cornea**. The cornea is a protective layer, a window, of sorts, that allows light to pass into the eye.

A thin layer of tissue called the **conjunctiva** attaches to the front part of the sclera and the eyelids. If you get a speck of dirt in your eye, you don't have to worry about it traveling to the back of your eyeball and getting stuck there because the conjunctiva prevents foreign objects from going very far. Tears keep the front of the eye and the conjunctiva moist and eventually wash away any foreign objects. Sometimes tear ducts become blocked or don't produce enough fluid, a condition called **dry eye syndrome** that causes the eye to become inflamed and irritated and can increase the risk of infection. When bacteria get into the folds between the conjunctiva and the eyelids, it can cause an infection called **conjunctivitis**, more commonly known as pinkeye. Dry eyes are not necessary for an infection to take hold, but it does increase the risk.

Just behind the cornea is a ring of colored tissue called the **iris**. This tissue gives the eyes their distinctive blue, green, or brown color, and the fibers within it are arranged like spokes in a wheel. The iris is a donut-shaped muscle that controls the amount of light that enters the eye by opening or closing the **pupil**, the black hole in the center of it. At night, when the light is dim, the pupil dilates to allow more light to enter the eye. For this reason, when you walk into a dark room, you may need a few seconds for your eyes to adjust. During the day, when the light is brighter, the pupil becomes smaller, allowing just enough light to enter for optimal vision. Too much light can be blinding, as you may have experienced by suddenly turning on the light in a dark room; at that point, your pupils are dilated, and although they respond quickly, enough light enters to blind you for a few seconds.

Just behind the pupil is the transparent and oval shaped **lens**. Its function is to focus incoming light onto the **retina**, the light-sensitive layer of nerve tissue that covers the inside surface of the eye. The **ciliary muscle** holds the lens in place. It contracts and relaxes to change the shape of the elastic-like lens, which can bulge to increase it curvature or stretch and become thinner and flatter. A flatter lens allows us to see distant objects while a fatter, more curved lens, allows us to focus up close. The process by which the lens changes its optical power to maintain a clear image or focus on an object at various distances is call **accommodation**.

As we age, changes often occur in the lens that can interfere with vision. In most people, the lens is transparent and elastic so that it is capable of changing shape and directing light to the retina. Overexposure to ultraviolet (UV) light from the sun and other sources of oxidative stress can cause the lens to harden and become milky, creating a common condition known as **cataracts**.

Fluids fill the spaces inside the eyeball. These are very important, for they help the eyeball to maintain its shape, direct light rays to the retina, and circulate nutrients to the cells within the eye. When light enters the eye, it passes through the cornea and travels through a space called the **anterior chamber**, which is filled with a fluid called **aqueous humor;** *humor* has nothing to do with being funny in this case, as it is Latin for "fluid." The light continues its journey through the pupil and then through the lens. As the light exits the lens, it passes into another chamber in the center of the eye, the **posterior chamber**, which is filled with a fluid called **vitreous humor.** Aqueous and vitreous humor are derived from plasma, the clear fluid in blood, and are continually circulated in and out of the eye chambers, bringing in nutrients and carrying away waste. The vitreous humor is thicker or less watery than the aqueous humor.

Sometimes, the ducts that drain these fluids from the eye become clogged, and while fluid continues to enter the eye, it cannot easily exit. Consequently, pressure builds inside the eye and pushes against the blood vessels that feed the retina. Reduced blood flow causes the retina to degenerate, leading to progressive vision loss that could end in blindness. This condition is called **glaucoma**.

When light hits the retina at the back of the eye, the light energy is converted into electrical signals, which are sent to the brain by way of the **optic nerve**. These signals are then relayed to the visual cortex at the back of the brain and decoded into visual images that we can understand.

Most of the light that enters the eye is focused by the lens on a small area of the retina called the **macula**. At the center of the macula is a small depression, the **fovea**. The macula contains specialized cells for seeing fine detail. When you focus on something directly in front of you, such as these words you are reading, the macula allows you to distinguish each of the letters clearly. Light coming into the eye from the side strikes other parts of the retina, allowing you to see the periphery, but with less precision; this is why you can't read or distinguish fine details with your peripheral vision. Sometimes, in older people, the macula begins to degenerate leading to **age-related macular degeneration**. Macular degeneration affects central vision first and gradually progresses outward, to the periphery.

The retina contains microscopic light-sensitive or photoreceptor cells called **rods** and **cones**. Dim light can stimulate the rods, allowing us to see at night. Brighter light is needed to stimulate the cones, which are used for daytime vision and to see color. Rod cells outnumber cone cells by about 17 to 1; there are about 7 million cone cells and 120 million rod cells in the retina. There are three kinds of cones, each of

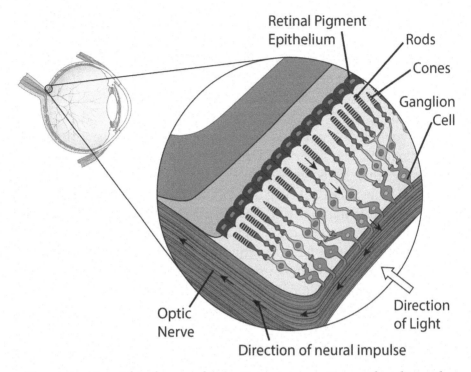

Retinal Pigment Epithelium

Rods

Cones

Ganglion Cell

Optic Nerve

Direction of Light

Direction of neural impulse

The retina is a thin layer of transparent nerve tissue that lines the inside of the eyeball. It is something like a layer cake, with each layer comprised of different types of cells. The outermost layer of photoreceptor cells (rod and cones) transmits a light-induced signal to the other nerve layers, down to the ganglion cell layer. Ganglion cells have long tails, axons, which extend from the retina and join together to form the optic nerve—a million-fiber cable that conveys visual information from the eye to the brain. Adjacent to the photoreceptor cells is a single layer of cells called retinal pigment epithelial cells (REP). Among other things, these perform the crucial function of absorbing and recycling the debris shed from the photoreceptor cells.

which are stimulated by a different color of light: red, green, or blue. These primary colors allow us to distinguish between all the different colors we see around us. Full-spectrum light, the colorless light from the sun, is a combination of all the different colors of light. Each color has a different wavelength. After rain, sunlight can be refracted by moisture in the atmosphere, which separates the different wavelengths to form a rainbow.

The range of light a human can see is called **visible light** and consists of wavelengths between 400 and 700 nanometers (nm). A nm is one billionth of a meter, so the wavelengths are incredibly small.

When full-spectrum light hits an object, such as a red "STOP" sign, the sign absorbs all the wavelengths of light except those around 650 nm (red). This wavelength of light is reflected off the sign and travels to your eyes, where it activates cone cells sensitive to 650 nm wavelength. As mentioned, each color has its own wavelength; for example, blue is about 460 nm, and green is about 520 nm. When we perceive a colored object, what we see is that part of the light spectrum that is not absorbed by the object but is reflected back into our eyes. Combinations of the three primary colors provide us with vision of all the different colors we sense in our environment.

Sunlight also contains wavelengths of light that our eyes cannot see because the cones in the human retina cannot pick them up. Ultraviolet light has wavelengths less than 400 nm, and infrared light has wavelengths larger than 700 nm, neither of which can be seen by the human eye. However, some animals can see these other colors. On the other hand, some animals don't have any color-sensitive cells and can only see various shades of black and white. Dogs, for example, have only two types of cone cells, so your friend Fido can see only combinations of yellow and blue. In contrast, many birds have four-color photoreceptors and can see ultraviolet light, as well as red, green, and blue. Butterflies have five-color photoreceptors. We have no idea what these other colors look like because we have no way to perceive them visually.

Some people are colorblind and cannot distinguish the difference between some colors in the human visual spectrum. Colorblindness is a genetic disorder that produces abnormal photopigments in the cones. Each of the three photopigments in the cones is sensitive to one of the primary colors of light. In many colorblind individuals, the green-sensitive photopigment is missing or deficient; in others the red-sensitive photopigment is abnormal. A deficiency of the blue-sensitive photopigment is very rare. Colorblindness may be a misleading term, as colorblind individuals still see colors, but they may not be able to distinguish between some. Although colorblindness is an abnormality, it is not considered a disability or disease.

Any damage to the retina can seriously affect vision. Even if the lens and all the other parts of the eye are working perfectly and focusing light directly on the retina, if the retina is not functioning properly, vision will be impaired at various levels of severity. Some health conditions that affect circulation, such as diabetes and atherosclerosis, can damage tiny blood vessels that feed the retina, leading to retinopathy (disease of the retina). The most common of these is **diabetic retinopathy**.

When light hits the rods and cones in the retina, an electric signal is created. This signal is sent to a layer of **ganglion cells** on the inner side of the retina. Ganglion cells have long **axons** (arms) that extend all the way to the brain. The signal is carried by the axons to the back of the eye, where they come together to form the optic nerve. The optic nerve exits the eye through the **optic disc**. There are no rods or cones in the area of the retina that forms the optic disc, and this produces a blind spot in our field of vision; blind spots are off center, so they do not interfere with central vision, and the spot is in a different part of your visual field for each eye. When both eyes are open, the opposite eye compensates for the blind spot in the other. When you close one eye, your brain compensates to fill the void. Ordinarily, you would never know you have a blind spot, however, you can locate it. See the box below to find your blind spot.

How to Find Your Blind Spot

To find your blind spot, take a piece of white paper and draw a small X on the right side. Using a ruler, measure about 5 inches (12 cm) to the left of the X and draw a black 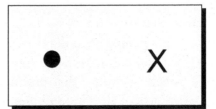 dot about the size of a penny. Hold the paper in front of you, at arm's length, close your right eye, and focus on the X with your left eye. You should see the black dot with your peripheral vision. Slowly move the paper toward your face. As you do so, the dot will disappear at a certain distance, but it will reappear as you bring the paper closer to your face. The area where the dot disappears is the blind spot in your left eye.

REFRACTIVE ERRORS

Chances are you wear glasses. Most people living in affluent countries do. Eyeglasses are used to correct refractive errors. Refraction is the bending of light as it passes through one object and into another. In the eye, light rays are bent (refracted) as they pass through the cornea and the lens. The light is then focused on the retina. Focusing a clear image on the retina is essential for good vision, for if the incoming light does not focus precisely onto the retina, vision becomes blurred.

Fortunately, most refractive errors are easy to correct. In areas of the world where medical care is readily available, most people with refractive errors have their vision corrected with a pair of prescription eyeglasses or contact lenses. In areas without adequate medical services or where people cannot afford proper medical care, refractive errors often go uncorrected.

Refractive errors occur when the shape of the eye prevents light from focusing directly on the retina. The length of the eyeball changes the shape or curve of the cornea, shortening or lengthening the focal point of rays of light that pass through to the retina. For reasons not fully understood, the eyeball is often not perfectly shaped, which leads to these problems.

In a normal eye, light rays enter the eye and come together into a clear focus on the retina. The image is inverted when it hits the

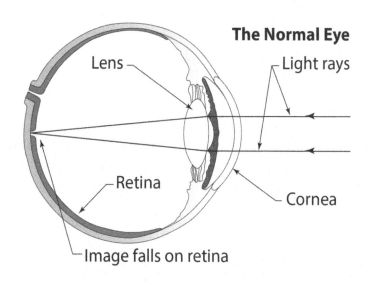

The Normal Eye

Lens

Light rays

Retina

Cornea

Image falls on retina

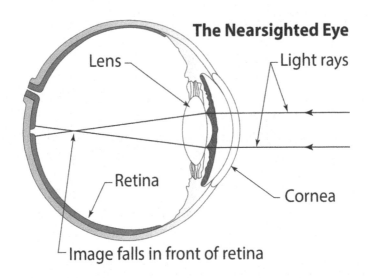

The Nearsighted Eye

Lens

Light rays

Retina

Cornea

Image falls in front of retina

retina, but the brain easily rights the image; otherwise, we would see everything upside down. However, the brain cannot correct an image that is not sharply focused. If our eyeball is elongated, the image focuses in front of the retina rather than on it. The rays of light the retina receives are slightly out of focus, producing a blurry image. This condition is called myopia, or nearsightedness. A person with myopia can see objects that are up close clearly, but objects that are far away appear blurry.

If the eyeball is shorter than normal, the light focuses behind the retina, also producing a blurry image. This condition is called hyperopia, or farsightedness. A person who is farsighted can see distant objects clearly but not those that are up close. However, people experience hyperopia differently. Some people may not notice any problems with their vision, especially when they are young. For people with significant hyperopia, vision can be blurry for objects at any distance, near or far.

As we age, the eye lens begins to lose some of its natural elasticity so it can no longer change shape enough to bring near objects into sharp focus. This loss of close vision is called presbyopia, sometimes referred to as "oldsightedness." Presbyopia often becomes noticeable around the age of 40. Corrective lenses can help correct near-vision loss. This is why many older people need reading glasses or bifocals, if they have other refractive errors. Bifocals consist of two prescription

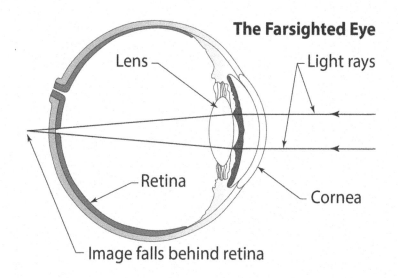

The Farsighted Eye

Lens

Light rays

Retina

Cornea

Image falls behind retina

lenses; the upper part of the lens may be needed for nearsightedness and the lower part for presbyopia.

Irregularities in the shape of the cornea or lens can interfere with the path of incoming light, causing the image to be distorted or fuzzy. This condition is called astigmatism. Like other refractive errors, astigmatism can be corrected with glasses or contact lenses.

Refractive errors can be identified during a comprehensive eye exam, which will include the reading an eye chart. Most refractive errors can be compensated for with corrective lenses, though surgery is an option in some cases. Refractive surgery aims to change the shape of the cornea permanently. This change in eye shape restores the focusing power of the eye by allowing light rays to focus more precisely on the retina for improved vision. Lasik is a popular form of refractive surgery in which the cornea is reshaped to change its optical power. In this type of surgery, the outer layer of the cornea is cut and raised up, then a laser is used to cut and flatten the underlying tissue. The outer flap of tissue is then replaced and allowed to heal. Lasik surgery can be used to correct nearsightedness, farsightedness, and astigmatism.

Refractive errors are the most common of all visual problems. According to the Vision Council of America, approximately 75 percent of adults use some type of vision correction. About 64 percent of them wear eyeglasses, and about 11 percent wear contact lenses.

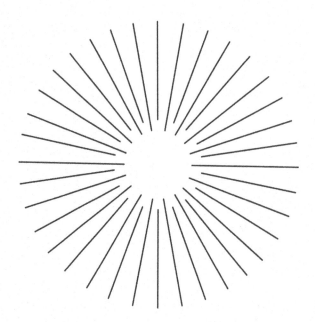

Self-test for astigmatism. Cover one eye and focus your sight at the center of the wheel. If any of the lines appear darker or thicker than the others, you have astigmatism. Test each eye.

Over half of all women and about 42 percent of men wear glasses. Similarly more women than men wear contacts, 18 percent and 14 percent respectively.

Approximately 30 percent of the American population is nearsighted, and about 60 percent is farsighted. It is likely that the percentages in Europe, Australia, and most other affluent countries are quite similar. The majority of young people who wear glasses are nearsighted, but as people age, they are more likely to need vision correction for farsightedness and presbyopia. About 25 percent of people who wear glasses to see at a distance will end up needing reading glasses or bifocals as they get older. About one-third of the people who wear glasses have astigmatism in one or both eyes.

A number of books have been written on vision therapy, a system of eye exercises and relaxation techniques designed to improve vision affected by refractive errors and reduce the need for glasses. You may have seen ads claiming to miraculously improve eyesight to the point that you will be able to throw away your glasses. Vision therapy was introduced by a New York ophthalmologist by the name of William H.

Bates (1860-1931). He developed the Bates Method for better eyesight, and in 1920, he published a book titled *Perfect Sight Without Glasses*. Many of the principles on which he based his theory were at odds with the conventional medical beliefs at the time, and they are still just as controversial today. In 1943, 12 years after Bates's death, a revised edition of his book was published under the title *Better Eyesight Without Glasses*. That edition contained no photographs, and some of the more controversial theories were removed. The Bates Method does offer some useful techniques, although it isn't the miracle cure it is often portrayed as in advertisements. A form of vision therapy is practiced today among some optometrists. It can be helpful in cases of strabismus, lazy eye, poor visual perception, accommodation, and, to some extent, refractive errors and can be used in conjunction with the methods discussed in this book. Bates's original book is now in the public domain, and you can download a free copy by going to http://www.iblindness.org/ebooks/perfect-sight-without-glasses/.

While vision therapy can be helpful, we will not cover that topic in this book. Rather, we will discuss how you can use diet and nutrition to prevent and correct visual impairment caused by common eye diseases that rob people of their eyesight.

VISUAL IMPAIRMENT

Most of us have experienced reading the letters on a Snellen chart when taking an eye examine (see illustration on the following page). The first line consists of a single large letter, which may be one of several letters, for example E, H, or N. Subsequent rows have increasing numbers of letters that decrease in size. The person taking the test covers one eye and, from a distance of 20 feet (6 m), reads aloud the letters of each row, beginning at the top. The smallest row that can be read accurately indicates the visual acuity in that eye. Since visual acuity can differ in each eye, the test is repeated with the other eye.

People with normal vision are able to read Line 8 on the chart; this is referred to as 20/20 (6/6) vision. If the smallest readable letters are larger (Lines 1 to 7), vision is designated as the distance from the chart (20 feet) over the distance corresponding to the smallest letter that can be read. For example, a person who can only read down to

Line 2 has a visual acuity of 20/100. This means a person would have to stand 20 feet from an object to see it with the same degree of clarity as a normally sighted person could from 100 feet.

In most cases, corrective lenses can improve vision to 20/20. However, in some cases this is not possible. Eyesight that cannot be improved to at least 20/70 with corrective lenses is referred to as "low vision." When a person has low vision, he or she is considered visually impaired. If your eyesight is poor, 20/200 or worse, but can be corrected to better than 20/70 with eyeglasses, you are not considered visually impaired.

Snellen chart.

Low vision describes visual clarity from 20/70 to 20/200 with corrective lenses; anyone with worse sight is considered legally blind, even though many would think that blindness refers to people who can see nothing at all, not even shades of light. On the contrary, most people who are classified as legally blind do have some limited sight or can see shades of light, shapes, colors, or objects. Only about 10 percent of those people who are legally blind have no vision whatsoever.

The Snellen chart only measures the clarity or sharpness of a person's central vision. However, we do not see just straight ahead, but from the side as well, even when our eyes are directed forward. This is our peripheral vision. The entire area of vision is called the visual field. Some people have good central vision but poor peripheral vision or have no vision (blind spots) in parts of their visual field.

The normal visual field is about 170 degrees, but the loss of peripheral vision results in a narrowing of this field. A person can be legally blind even if they have a normal degree of clarity straight ahead but a visual field of less than 20 degrees (side vision that is so reduced that it appears as if the person is looking through a tunnel).

Currently, the estimated number of visually impaired people in the world is 285 million (1 out of every 25), 39 million blind and 246 million having low vision; 65 percent of people are visually impaired, and 82 percent of all blind are 50 years or older.[1]

According to the World Health Organization (WHO), the most common causes of blindness around the world, in order of prevalence, are:

- Cataracts
- Glaucoma
- Age-related macular degeneration
- Corneal opacities
- Diabetic retinopathy
- Childhood blindness (genetic defects and nutritional deficiencies)
- Uncorrected refractive errors
- Trachoma
- Onchocerciasis

Visual impairment is a much greater problem in developing counties than in developed countries. According to the WHO, 90 percent of blind people live in the developing world. Of these, cataracts are the most common cause. Equally as common are uncorrected refractive errors, which are generally easily corrected with eyeglasses. Serious eye infections, such as trachoma (bacteria) and onchocerciasis (parasite) are a big problem in some areas of the world where medical care is unavailable or inadequate. Corneal opacities, or clouding of the cornea, may develop from injury, infection, or a variety of less common and usually genetic syndromes. In developed countries where eyeglasses, cataract surgery, and medications are more readily available, age-related macular degeneration, glaucoma, and diabetic retinopathy are the leading causes of blindness.

Other causes of vision loss include:

- Accidents
- Blocked blood vessels (atherosclerosis)
- Complications of premature birth (retrolental fibroplasia)
- Complications of eye surgery
- Lazy eye
- Optic neuritis
- Stroke
- Retinitis pigmentosa
- Tumors such as retinoblastoma and optic glioma

3

Common Eye Disorders

CATARACTS

Cataract is the leading cause of visual impairment throughout the world and is responsible for over 50 percent of all cases of blindness. Risk of developing cataract increases with age and poses a serious threat to the elderly, with approximately 25 percent of those over 65 years and 50 percent over 80 years of age experiencing a serious loss of vision as a result of it. Everyone is potentially at risk of developing cataract. It is so common in the elderly that it is often considered a normal part of the aging process; however, people can and do live long lives without ever experiencing this condition. Although cataract usually surfaces sometime after the age of 60, some people develop it in their 40s and 50s. In the United States, cataract affects 1 out of every 14 people age 40 and over.

Surgery is the standard treatment for this condition, and 1.35 million cataract operations are performed in the United States every year. Worldwide, 18 million people are blind because of cataracts.[1] Although cataracts can be successfully treated with surgery, in many countries people cannot afford the treatment, are unaware of it, or do not have access to appropriate medical services. As a consequence, the disease usually progresses untreated, resulting in the high incidence of blindness seen worldwide.

Cataract is caused by clouding of the normally transparent lens inside the eye. The cloudy lens obstructs light from passing though and focusing on the retina at the back of the eye, interfering with vision. Initially, cataract may be so subtle and come on so slowly that it is not noticed. As time goes on, vision can grow increasingly hazy. Cataract usually affects both eyes, yet each eye can progress at a different rate. Those with cataracts often experience difficulty in reading, driving, recognizing faces and objects, and coping with glare from bright lights.

The most common symptoms associated with cataracts are:

- Cloudy or blurry vision
- Colors begin to fade
- Glare or a halo appearance around lights
- Poor night vision
- Double vision or multiple images in one eye
- Frequent prescription changes in corrective lenses

These symptoms can also be a sign of other eye problems. If you have any of these symptoms, check with your eye doctor.

Cataract is classified according to its location in the lens. Nuclear cataract forms in the center of the lens, directly behind the pupil and can interfere significantly with vision. Cortical cataract occurs on the outer edges of the lens, and posterior subcapular cataract forms near the back of the lens, right in the path of light on its way to the retina. Posterior subcapular cataract interferes with reading, reduces vision in bright light, and causes glare or halos around lights at night.

In a small number of cases cataracts can be caused by genetic defects, infection, or injury. In the vast majority of cases, however, the characteristic clouding is the result of damage caused by oxidation and glycation—processes that produce destructive free radicals. In age-related cataracts the clouding is due to natural proteins and lipids (fats) in the lens becoming denatured or degraded. This degradation is caused by chemical reactions from free radicals and advanced glycation end products (AGEs). Normally, the eyes contain antioxidant enzymes that protect them from destructive free-radical reactions. However, if the diet is poor in antioxidant nutrients and exposure to environmental factors that promote free-radical generation is excessive, delicate eye tissue can become damaged. Factors that promote free-radical generation include exposure to environmental toxins, cigarette smoke, pollution, ultraviolet light, radiation from medical equipment, and certain drugs and foods. Corticosteroids, for instance, are known to induce cataract development.[2]

People with diabetes are 60 percent more likely to develop cataracts than the general population. They also tend to get cataracts at a younger age, and the condition progresses faster. High blood sugar associated with diabetes accelerates the production of AGEs, which undoubtedly affects the occurrence and progression of the disease.

Ultraviolet (UV) radiation from the sun can initiate free-radical reactions in our skin and eyes. Just as overexposure to the sun can redden and burn our skin, it can also damage our eyes. For this reason, doctors often recommend that patients wear ultraviolet-blocking sunglasses when they go outdoors.

Antioxidant supplements such as vitamins A, C, and E, as well as lutein and zeaxanthin, are often recommended as protection against cataracts because they help to clean up free radicals. N-acetylcarnosine, a naturally occurring antioxidant found in a variety of human tissues, is believed to be effective in quenching free radicals that promote cataracts. Studies have shown it to be particularly active against oxidation in the different parts of the lens of the eye.[3-4] N-acetylcarnosine is included in a number of eyedrops intended for the treatment of cataracts.

When cataracts greatly interfere with vision, the damaged lens can be surgically removed and replaced with an artificial one. This surgery involves numbing the eye with an anesthetic. A cut is then made through the clear cornea to allow access to the lens. A needle or small pair of forceps is used to create a circular hole in the capsule in which the lens sits. A probe is used to break up and emulsify the lens into a liquid, which is then sucked away. If the cataract is severe and the lens too hard to emulsify, it must be cut out and removed manually, and a flexible plastic lens is inserted in its place. The final step is to inject salt water into the corneal wound to cause the area to swell and seal the incision. If cataracts affect both eyes, surgery is performed on one eye at a time, four to eight weeks apart. About 90 percent of surgery patients can achieve a corrected vision of 20/40 or better after surgery.

While cataract surgery is relatively safe, the rate of associated complications is significant. Opacification, clouding of the posterior lens capsule, occurs in 30 to 50 percent of patients within 2 years of cataract removal and requires laser treatment. A further 0.8 percent experience retinal detachments, approximately 1 percent are re-hospitalized for corneal problems, and about 0.1 percent develop endophthalmitis, severe inflammation usually caused by infection. In addition, those with diabetes have an increased risk of developing diabetic retinopathy and glaucoma as a result of surgery. Although the risks are small, the large number of procedures performed means that 26,000 individuals develop serious complications as a result of cataract surgery annually in the United States alone. Therefore, caution should be taken when making a decision to undergo this procedure.

GLAUCOMA

Next to cataracts, glaucoma is the most common cause of blindness worldwide. It is estimated that 60 million people, 1 out of every 120, have glaucoma. The disease can occur at any age, however, older people are at highest risk, but babies can be born with it, and approximately 1 out of every 10,000 in the United States are. Young adults can also develop glaucoma.

A normal, healthy eye is filled with a fluid in an amount that is carefully regulated to maintain the shape of the eyeball. In glaucoma, the balance of this fluid is disturbed. Fluid enters the eye more rapidly than it leaves, and pressure inside the eyeball, called intraocular pressure, builds up. The pressure pinches the veins and arteries that carry blood to and from the retina and optic nerve. Vision is gradually lost because the retina and nerve are damaged. Generally, there is no pain, nor are there any obvious symptoms. Peripheral vision is affected first, and vision loss may be so gradual that it is initially unnoticeable. As the disease progresses, side vision decreases, and the field of view narrows into tunnel vision. If left untreated, the pressure will permanently damage the optic nerve, causing complete blindness.

Glaucoma is often called the "sneak thief of sight" because it creeps up without warning and by the time it is detected, substantial vision may already be lost. Since there are few symptoms in the early stages, many people have the disease without knowing it. It is estimated that as many as half of those with glaucoma are not even aware of it. Symptoms are subtle, but there may be some hazy vision and mild discomfort in the eye and, later, a barely noticeable loss of peripheral vision. As the disease progresses, there is reduced visual acuity, and greatly increased fluid pressure can cause the appearance of colored rings or halos around bright objects. Glaucoma can develop in one or both eyes. There are a number of reasons why intraocular pressure builds up in the eye: inflammation and swelling narrowing the drainage ducts, clogging the ducts with debris from the eye (e.g., a fragment of iris tissue), chronic high blood pressure, and injury caused by trauma, just to name a few.

In some rare cases, a child can be born with a defect of the eye that slows the normal drainage of fluid, a condition known as congenital glaucoma. Affected children usually have obvious symptoms, such as cloudy eyes, sensitivity to light, and excessive tearing. Conventional surgery is the suggested treatment, because medicines are not effective and can cause more serious side effects in infants and be difficult to administer. If done properly, surgery provides children with a good chance of having normal vision.

Secondary glaucoma can develop as a complication of other medical conditions. For example, a severe form of glaucoma called neovascular glaucoma can result from poorly controlled diabetes or heart disease. Other types of glaucoma sometimes occur with cataracts, certain eye tumors, or a condition called uveitis (inflammation of tissues encapsulating the eyeball). Glaucoma sometimes develops after other eye surgeries or serious eye injuries. Steroids used to treat eye inflammations and other diseases can trigger glaucoma in some people.

In some cases, the cause is unknown. One form of the disease occurs in people with normal eye pressure, a condition known as low- or normal-tension glaucoma. Lowering eye pressure with the use of medication slows the disease in some people but may worsen it in others.

Early detection and treatment can often protect the eyes against serious vision loss. Glaucoma can be detected by a visual field test that measures peripheral vision, by measuring the pressure inside the eye using an instrument called a tonometer, by measuring the thickness of the cornea, or by examining the retina and optic nerve though a special magnifying lens.

There is no medically recognized cure for glaucoma. Treatment focuses primarily on reducing intraocular pressure and may include

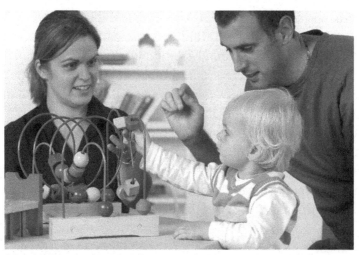

Normal vision.

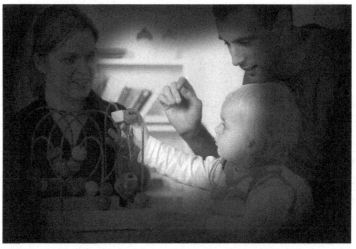

Glaucoma. There may be tunnel vision and missing areas of vision.

medicines, laser therapy, surgery, or a combination of any of these. While these treatments may save remaining vision, they do not recover sight that has already been lost due to glaucoma. This is why early diagnosis is very important.

Medicines, in the form of eyedrops or pills, are the most common early treatment for glaucoma. Taken regularly, they can lower eye pressure. Some medicines cause the eye to make less fluid, and others lower pressure by helping fluid drain from the eye. Some medicines may cause headaches, stinging, burning, or redness in the eyes. Because glaucoma often has no symptoms, people may be tempted to stop taking their medication or even forget, but these medicines must be taken regularly, without interruption, as directed, to preserve eyesight.

In more advanced stages of the disease, laser or conventional surgery may be performed to open the ducts that allow fluid to better drain from the eyes. Unfortunately, approximately 10 percent of people who receive proper treatment still experience loss of vision.

MACULAR DEGENERATION

As the name of this disease implies, the macula, the part of the retina responsible for sharp forward vision, degenerates, causing a loss of central vision in the affected eye. When the macula is damaged, the center of the field of view may appear blurry, distorted, or dark.

The macula begins to degenerate in one out of every four people over the age of 65, and in one out of every three people over the age of 80. It affects over 30 million people worldwide.

There are different forms of the disease. The most common, age-related macular degeneration (AMD), usually appears sometime after the age of 50. This condition is the leading cause of blindness in persons over the age of 65. When you hear macular degeneration being discussed, it most often refers to this form of the disease. Another far less common form of the disease occurs in younger people called Stargardt disease. This is a hereditary disease caused by a chromosome defect. It usually appears sometime between the ages of 6 and 20 and is marked by a rapid loss of visual acuity.

There are two forms of AMD, dry and wet. The dry form accounts for 90 percent of cases and is characterized by the gradual wearing out of the retinal pigment cells in the macula. Although visual acuity loss usually does not progress beyond the 20/200 level, this is still a significant disability. Currently, there is no known medical treatment that can prevent, stop, or reverse this form of macular degeneration. Care is focused on teaching the patient to cope with the condition and make the most out of what vision remains, such as reading large-print books, the help of a magnifying glass, and ensuring that lighting is adequate whenever detail work is necessary.

The wet form AMD is characterized by an abnormal growth of a network of tiny blood vessels within or very close to the macula. These vessels cause leakage of blood and fluid beneath the macula, resulting in distorted, blurred vision. This form of macular degeneration can cause complete loss of central vision; therefore, it is potentially more serious than the dry form. Fortunately, laser therapy can seal off the leaking blood vessels and help prevent further vision loss. If diagnosed and treated early, when the blood vessel network is small, significant loss of central vision may be avoided.

In some people, AMD advances so slowly that vision loss does not occur for a long time. In others, the disease progresses faster and may lead to a significant loss of vision in one or both eyes. As AMD progresses, a blurred area near the center of vision is a common symptom. Over time, the blurred area may grow, or you may develop blank spots in your central vision that might interfere with simple, everyday activities, such as the ability to see faces, drive, read, write, or do close work, including cooking.

Not every case of early-stage AMD will degrade into a more severe or late stage. For people who have early AMD in one eye and

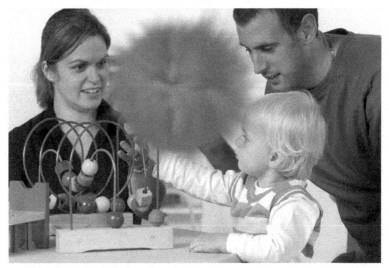

Macular degeneration. Side vision is normal, but central vision is slowly lost.

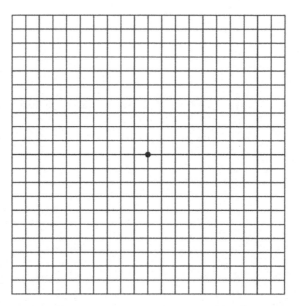

The Amsler grid is often used to test for macular degeneration. To test yourself, wear reading glasses if you need them, and place the grid at the normal distance where you would place any reading material. Cover one eye, then focus on the dot in the center. Do any of the lines look wavy, blurred, or distorted? If your sight is normal, all lines should be straight, all intersections should form right angles, and all the squares should be the same size. An example of a distorted image can be seen on the following page. Test the other eye.

no signs of AMD in the other, about 5 percent will develop advanced AMD after 10 years. For those who have early AMD in both eyes, about 14 percent will develop late AMD in at least one eye after 10 years.

If you have late AMD in one eye only, you may not notice any changes in your overall vision. As long as your other eye is seeing clearly, you may still be able to drive, read, and see fine details. However, late AMD in one eye means you are at increased risk for late AMD in the other. If you notice distortion or blurred vision, even if it doesn't seem to affect your daily life much, it would be wise to consult with an eye care professional.

Early AMD has few noticeable symptoms. Although AMD is usually diagnosed in older people, the disease starts at a much younger

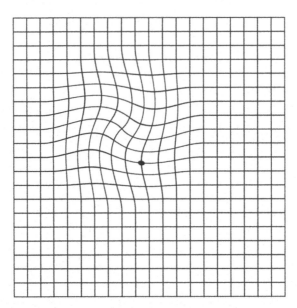

The Amsler grid as might be seen by a person with macular degeneration.

age and slowly progresses. The only way to tell if you are developing AMD is through an examination, which may involve a visual acuity test with an eye chart, examining the back of the eye with a magnifying lens, or looking at an Amsler grid. The Amsler grid is a quick and easy way to evaluate central vision. For this test, patients are given a sheet of paper that contains a grid of horizontal and vertical lines. The patient is asked to note any distortion of the lines in the center of the grid. This test can be done at home and repeated periodically. If distortion is seen in the grid, this still does not necessarily indicate AMD, but it does reveal some kind of central vision distortion, and further testing is needed to come to a definite diagnosis.

Medical treatment for AMD is limited. However, researchers have found connections between the disease and lifestyle. Smoking, high blood pressure, obesity, and the excessive consumption of sugar and polyunsaturated vegetable oils increase risk. On the other hand, regular exercise and a healthy diet with ample vitamins, minerals, and antioxidants reduce the risk. Adopting healthy habits may delay or even prevent the disease.

DIABETIC RETINOPATHY

Diabetes is a lifelong, progressive disease caused by the body's inability to produce insulin or use insulin to its full potential. It is characterized by chronically elevated blood glucose levels. Diabetes affects the cardiovascular system, causing the circulatory system to degenerate. This leads to many complications, such as heart attacks, strokes, kidney failure, peripheral neuropathy, and retinopathy. In the United States, Europe, and Australia, diabetic retinopathy is the leading cause of blindness in individuals age 20 to 65.

Diabetic retinopathy is a general term for all disorders of the retina caused by diabetes. Poorly controlled diabetes can initiate changes in the blood vessels in the retina that can lead to severe vision loss and blindness. Both eyes are usually affected. There are two major types of diabetic retinopathy: nonproliferative and proliferative.

Nonproliferative retinopathy is the most common. It occurs when capillaries in the back of the eye balloon and form pouches. These ballooned blood vessels leak fluid and blood at the macula, where focusing occurs. When the macula swells with fluid, vision blurs and can be lost entirely.

Nonproliferative retinopathy can progress into the more serious proliferative retinopathy. As the tiny blood vessels swell and become damaged, new blood vessels begin to grow along the retina to take their place. These new vessels are abnormal and fragile and can leak blood, blocking vision. Injury from the damaged blood vessels can also cause scar tissue to develop. As the scar tissue begins to heal, it shrinks, which can distort the retina or pull it out of place, a condition called retinal detachment.

The longer a person has diabetes, the more likely they are to develop retinopathy. Almost everyone with type 1 diabetes and most of those with type 2 will eventually develop nonproliferative retinopathy. Between 40 to 45 percent of those diagnosed with diabetes already have some stage of retinopathy. The more serious proliferative retinopathy is far less common.

Both nonproliferative and proliferative retinopathy can develop without any noticeable symptoms, as the retina can be damaged before the person notices any change in vision. Even in cases of proliferative retinopathy, people sometimes have no symptoms until permanent damage has occurred. Blurred vision may occur when the macula swells from leaking fluid. At first, a few specks of blood or spots may also interfere with vision. These spots sometimes clear without treatment, allowing the person to see more clearly; however, bleeding can reoccur. If it advances to the proliferative stage, risk of permanent vision loss is high. Diabetics should have comprehensive eye exams at least once a year. People with proliferative retinopathy can reduce their risk of blindness by 95 percent with timely treatment and appropriate follow-up care.

Diabetic retinopathy is treated with laser surgery. A procedure called focal laser treatment is used to treat nonproliferative retinopathy. The doctor places up to several hundred small laser burns in the areas of retinal leakage surrounding the macula. These burns slow the leakage and reduce the amount of fluid in the retina. The surgery is usually completed in one session, though a patient may need multiple treatments to control the leaking fluid.

Proliferative retinopathy is treated with a procedure called scatter laser treatment. Scatter laser treatment helps to shrink the abnormal blood vessels. The doctor places 1,000 to 2,000 laser burns in the areas of the retina away from the macula, causing the abnormal blood

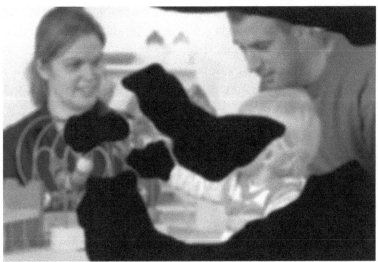

Diabetic retinopathy. Vision may be blurred, there may be shadows or missing areas of vision, and difficultly seeing at night.

vessels to shrink. Because a high number of laser burns is necessary, two or more sessions are usually required to complete treatment. Although scatter laser treatment may slightly reduce side vision, color vision, and night vision, treatment can save the rest of the patient's sight.

Neither type of laser treatment is a cure, but they can significantly reduce (but rarely stop) further vision loss. Once you develop diabetic retinopathy, especially proliferative retinopathy, you will always be at risk for new bleeding and may need periodic follow-up treatments.

Bringing blood sugar under control, through a proper diet, is the best treatment for diabetes and reduces the risk of all related complications, including retinopathy.

OPTIC NEURITIS

Optic neuritis is defined as inflammation of the optic nerve. Inflammation causes the optic nerve to swell, which can result in injury to the nerve fibers and partial loss of vision. Symptoms of optic neuritis may include blurred or double vision, pain, nystagmus (uncontrolled eye movements), loss of color vision, blind spots, and temporary blindness. Loss of vision usually occurs in only one eye and tends to worsen over the course of several days before getting better.

Double vision occurs when the pair of muscles that control particular eye movements are not coordinated due to weakness in one or more of the muscles. Although annoying, double vision usually resolves on its own without medical treatment. Vision typically returns to normal within 2 to 3 weeks without treatment. Treatment options are limited and usually involve oral or IV administration of steroids to calm inflammation.

The exact cause of optic neuritis is not known, however, it frequently occurs in people who suffer from other inflammatory illnesses such as lupus and sarcoidosis, as well as some infectious diseases such as Lyme disease and rubella. It is a common symptom of multiple sclerosis (MS). According to the National Multiple Sclerosis Society, 55 percent of people with MS will have an episode of optic neuritis. It is often the first sign of the disease. Optic neuritis associated with MS may last anywhere from 4 to 12 weeks.

People who develop optic neuritis without an associated disease, such as MS, have a good chance of complete recovery without a recurrence. Approximately 50 to 60 percent of people who experience optic neuritis, without an associated disease, eventually develop MS, and those with MS often experience repeat episodes.

STROKE

If an artery that feeds the brain becomes blocked or ruptures, the brain cells cannot get the nutrients and oxygen they need, causing them to die. This is called a stroke. Strokes can cause vision impairment when the resulting tissue damage occurs in one of the regions of the brain that process visual information. The majority of visual processing occurs in the occipital lobe, in the back of the brain. Most strokes affect only one side of the brain. If the right occipital lobe is injured, the left field of vision in each eye may be affected. A stroke in the left occipital lobe can affect the right field of vision in each eye. Rarely are both sides of the brain affected.

As many as one out of every four stroke survivors experiences vision loss. In most cases, vision loss is never fully recovered, although partial recovery is possible and usually occurs within the first months after the stroke.

The most common type of stroke-induced vision impairment is the loss of half of the field of vision; but vision loss may be restricted to a quarter of the visual field or to a blind spot within the field of vision. Other vision problems are also possible. The brain stem is the starting point for three pairs of nerves that control eye movements. A stroke in this area can result in only one eye moving correctly. This can cause double vision or the inability of both eyes to look in a particular direction. Visual stability may also be affected. For example, stationary objects may appear to move. As you might imagine, this can make reading or focusing difficult. The brain may have difficulty visually comprehending or recognizing familiar faces or objects. Loss of feeling and muscle control may occur around the eyes, making blinking difficult, not allowing an eyelid to properly close or sometimes causing a droopy lid.

Just as the brain can suffer a stroke, so can the eye itself, when the veins or arteries that feed the retina and optic nerve are blocked or ruptured. This is called an eye occlusion or an eye stroke. It occurs suddenly and generally involves only one eye. Depending on which veins or arteries are affected, eye occlusions can cause near or total loss of vision, loss of peripheral or central vision, distorted vision, or blind spots.

More than 80 percent of people who experience an eye stroke do recover most of their vision over a period of several months, although noticeable and permanent vision problems such as blind spots or distortions generally persist. Laser treatment, drugs, or surgery can shorten recovery time.

Most people who experience a stroke often have high blood pressure, atherosclerosis (plaque with hardening and narrowing of the arteries) or diabetes. Some have a combination of these and other disorders.

INFECTIONS

The two primary eye infections that result in the greatest number of cases of vision loss and blindness are trachoma and onchocerciasis. Trachoma is caused by the bacterium *Chlamydia trachomatis*. The disease progresses over a number of years, as repeated infections cause scarring on the inside of the eyelid. This has earned it the name of the "quiet disease." The eyelashes eventually turn in and rub on the cornea. The cornea becomes scarred as a result, leading to severe vision loss and eventually blindness. The disease is transmitted directly from eye to eye, mostly by flies, but it can also be spread by contact with an infected person's eyes or nose. The infection generally resolves on its own, but lack of proper sanitation, crowded living conditions, and not enough clean water and toilets leads to repeated infections. The World Health Organization estimates that 6 million people worldwide are blind due to trachoma, and another 150 million have active infections. It is most common in Africa, Asia, and Central and South America.

The trachoma bacterium is the most common cause of eye infections worldwide. In most cases, the infection is not recurrent or chronic, so it does not lead to permanent vision impairment and can be treated with antibiotics. The bacterium commonly inhabits the birth canal, therefore, antibiotics are often routinely applied to the eyes of newborns to prevent infection or conjunctivitis. In areas where sanitation and personal hygiene are better controlled, infections and serious complications are much less common.

Onchocerciasis, also known as river blindness, is the second most common cause of blindness due to infection. It is caused by a parasitic worm called *Onchocerica volvulus*. The worm is spread by bites from a black fly. Typically, many bites are required before infection occurs. Black flies live near rivers, which is why the disease is often called river blindness. Once inside a person, the worms create larva that make their way out of the skin, including the eye. Ninety-nine percent of cases occur in sub-Saharan Africa. There are drugs that can treat the disease.

Many microorganisms can infect the eyes, but not all are as dangerous, and most infections last only a few days. Conjunctivitis is a general term meaning inflammation of the conjunctiva, and it is characterized by red, itchy, watery eyes, thus, it is commonly called "pinkeye." Anything that causes inflammation in the conjunctiva can cause conjunctivitis. Infections are the usual suspects, but inflammation can also be caused by allergies, debris, or trauma.

OTHER CONDITIONS

There are numerous other disorders that affect the cornea, retina, and other parts of the eye. Some are genetic, while others are environmental or directly related to lifestyle. Since many degenerative eye conditions can creep up slowly without much warning, it is a good idea to visit your optometrist or ophthalmologist every three to five years for a comprehensive eye exam.

If you are age 60 or older, you should have a comprehensive eye exam at least every one to two years. In addition to cataracts, your eye doctor can check for signs of age-related macular degeneration, glaucoma, and other vision disorders. In many cases, early treatment of eye disease may save your sight.

4

Vision Busters

THE FREE RADICAL

What do all the following conditions have in common: cataracts, macular degeneration, glaucoma, diabetes, and Alzheimer's disease? You might say they are all associated with aging, but some can occur in the relatively young. The thing that ties all these conditions together, as well as most other degenerative disease, is free radicals. Free radicals, also known as reactive oxygen species (ROS), are renegade molecules that attack and destroy other molecules. Any tissue in our body is susceptible to free-radical damage, and the accumulation of this damage over many years results in degeneration of body tissues and loss of function, typifying the symptoms of old age.

Very simply, a free radical is a molecule with an unpaired electron in its outer orbit. The missing electron makes the molecule highly reactive and unstable. It aggressively seeks to steal an electron from a neighboring molecule. Once an electron is pulled away, the second molecule, now with one less electron, becomes a highly reactive free radical itself and pulls an electron off yet another nearby molecule. This process continues in a destructive chain reaction that may affect thousands of molecules.

Once a molecule becomes a free radical, its physical and chemical properties change in a process called oxidation. The normal function of such molecules is disrupted, affecting the entire cell of which they are a part. A living cell attacked by free radicals degenerates and becomes dysfunctional. Free radicals can attack our cells and literally rip their protective membranes apart. Sensitive cellular components like DNA, which carries the genetic blueprint of the cell, can be severely damaged in the process of oxidation.

Basically, oxidation is a process in which substances combine with oxygen or other nonmetallic elements in such a way as to cause degeneration. In the environment, this can be seen as rancidity of oils and hardening of rubber, but the classic example of free-radical deterioration in nature is that of rust. Iron exposed to the elements in the air readily oxidizes. In this process, the corroded iron expands, becomes brittle, and falls apart, due to disintegration or decay. When your body is attacked by free radicals, it essentially rusts and disintegrates, and the aging process is accelerated.

As cells are bombarded by free radicals, the tissues become progressively impaired. Some researchers believe free-radical destruction is the actual cause of aging. The older the body gets, the more damage it sustains from a lifetime of exposure to free radicals.

It appears that free radicals are at least partly to blame for the way we look, feel, and function as we get older. Free radicals slowly degenerate body tissues, and aging is a degenerative process. The effects of free-radical degeneration are, perhaps, most evident in our skin, specifically the collagen, which acts as the matrix that gives strength and flexibility to our tissues. Collagen is found everywhere in our bodies and holds everything together. It is what keeps our skin smooth, elastic, and youthful. When degraded by free radicals, the skin becomes dry, leathery, and wrinkled—all the classic signs of old age.

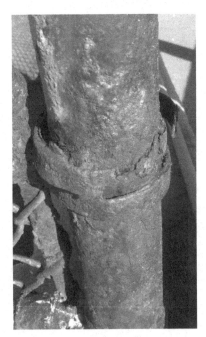

Tissues in the body attacked by free radicals degrade like this rusted metal fence post.

Free radicals affect the eyes in a similar manner. The white coating that forms on the lens in cataracts is a result of free-radical damage. The eyes, as well as the brain, are uniquely sensitive to oxidative injury because the cell membranes in these tissues contain a large percentage of highly vulnerable polyunsaturated fatty acids in concentrations among the highest in the body.

It is impossible to prevent all free-radical reactions that occur in the body, for they are part of everyday life. Free radicals form as a natural consequence of normal metabolic processes. The utilization of oxygen and glucose to produce energy produces free radicals as a byproduct. Every cell produces free radicals, but our cells are not left defenseless. Antioxidant enzymes are ever-present to quickly squelch these radicals before they can do too much damage.

In addition to the normal generation of free radicals inside our bodies, these rogue molecules are also produced by injury, infection, toxins, excessive stress, and various environmental stimuli. Diet is a major source of free radicals. Certain food additives, pesticide residue, chemicals, pollutants, and other toxins increase our free radical load. Free radical content can also be determined by the way food is cooked.

Polyunsaturated vegetable oils are one major source of free radicals in the diet. The polyunsaturated oils inside natural foods such as vegetables, nuts, and grains are not too much of a problem, so long as they are fresh, because nature always packages them with protective antioxidants to prevent rancidity (oxidation). It's when these oils are extracted and purified into liquid oils that they become troublesome. These oils spontaneously produce free radicals at room temperature. When they are heated, as in cooking, free-radical generation is greatly accelerated. Diets high in polyunsaturated vegetable oils can tremendously increase the body's free radical load. Polyunsaturated oils are so prone to free radical formation that the body's antioxidant reserves are quickly eaten up trying to neutralize them. Not only does this cause antioxidant deficiencies, but it also results in nutritional deficiencies as well, because many of these antioxidants are essential vitamins and minerals, crucial for good digestive function, hormone balance, a strong immune system, and proper eye function.

FREE RADICALS AND VISION LOSS

What do oxidation and free radicals have to do with vision loss? Lots! Free radicals are key players in the destructive processes that destroy delicate eye tissue, leading to cataracts, glaucoma, macular degeneration, diabetic retinopathy, and many other eye disorders.[1-4]

These common eye disorders generally surface later in life. For this reason, we refer to them as age-related cataracts or age-related macular degeneration, and so forth. While some of these conditions can and do occur in children, the number of these cases is very small in comparison to those in older adults. When these conditions do occur in children, it often involves genetics or gestational conditions. In adults, oxidative stress over the course of many years gradually breaks down eye tissue, leading to vision loss.

The longer we live, the greater our exposure to free radicals. After a lifetime of exposure to these destructive molecules, the eyes begin to degenerate. While age is a risk factor for many of these visual disorders, it is not the cause. Many people live long, healthy lives without ever developing any of these disorders. So why do some people develop cataracts or glaucoma and others do not? One of the primary reasons is excess exposure to oxidative stress; those people with the greatest exposure are at the greatest risk.

Free radicals are produced in our bodies every hour, every minute, and every second. In fact, they are continually produced inside each of our cells. The mitochondrion, the organelle in the cell that produces energy, generates free radicals as a byproduct of energy metabolism. These free radicals can cause substantial harm to the cell. In order to protect itself, the cell must maintain a reservoir of antioxidants on hand to extinguish these free radicals as quickly as possible so they do as little damage as possible. When this process is working as it should, the cells can live, function, divide, and propagate for a lifetime. This process may work smoothly for a long time, but over time, the cell wears out from repeated exposure to free radicals and eventually dies.

When this process is working as it should, the cells can provide a lifetime of trouble-free service. However, if antioxidant reserves become depleted or if free-radical formation speeds up and overwhelms the available antioxidants, free radical-induced damage can accelerate, causing the cells to prematurely age and die. If cells in your lens degenerate or die, the lens loses its elasticity and begins to develop white spots that interfere with vision. If any of the cells in the retina, the cones, rods, or ganglions are damaged or die, electrical impulses cannot be transmitted to the brain, and the result is vision loss. When cells that make up the many capillaries and blood vessels in the eye die, the vessels break and become leaky, and eyesight is compromised.

Free-radical damage is involved in all common eye disorders, if not as the primary cause, at least as a significant contributing factor. While free radicals are produced as a natural consequence of normal metabolic processes within our cells, their number and lifespan are determined, to a great extent, by our lifestyle choices. Diet, nutritional status, physical activity, environmental toxins, tobacco use, pollution, and excessive exposure to ultraviolet and other forms of radiation all have a dramatic effect the amount of oxidative stress we experience in our lives.

This means you don't have to be a helpless victim to degenerative eye disease. You can take an active role in stopping one of the central processes involved in visual degeneration. Through wise lifestyle choices, you can stop further degeneration and provide your body with the things it needs to heal and recover and possibly regain some or all of your lost vision.

*AGE*ING EYES
Advanced Glycation End Products (AGEs)

Oxidation isn't the only destructive force associated with aging and vision loss. Oxygen is a very reactive molecule and readily causes oxidation and free-radical generation. Likewise, glucose can react in a similar manner to cause glycation. This process is essentially the same as oxidation, except that glucose takes the place of the oxygen; to glycate something is to combine it with glucose. Like oxidation, glycation of proteins and polyunsaturated fats produces free radicals and other highly reactive and destructive molecular entities.

Glucose is a very sticky substance and combines easily with other molecules. It can stick to fats but is especially attracted to proteins. The glycation of proteins forms what are called advanced glycation end products (AGEs).

The effects of advanced glycation end products are aptly expressed in the acronym "AGE" because they literally age the body. Aging can be defined as the accumulation of damaged cells, and the more AGEs you have in your body, the "older" you become functionally, regardless of how many years you've lived. AGEs adversely affect other molecules, generating free radicals, oxidizing LDL cholesterol (thus creating the type of cholesterol that collects in arteries and promotes atherosclerosis, heart attacks, and strokes), degrading collagen (the major supporting structure in our organs and skin), damaging nerve tissue (including the brain and eyes), and wreaking havoc on just about every organ in the body. As we age, AGEs accumulate in the cornea, lens, vitreous humor, and retina. They are known to play an important role in the chronic complications of diabetes and in the development of diabetic retinopathy, macular degeneration, glaucoma, and cataracts,[5-7] as well as Alzheimer's and other neurodegenerative diseases.[8-10]

The AGEing hypothesis of aging was prompted by multiple observations that aged tissues are characterized by the accumulation of a variety of AGE products. AGEs are involved in a vicious cycle of inflammation, generation of free radicals, amplified production of AGEs, more inflammation, and so on.

We all experience the effects of AGEs to some extent; it is, unfortunately, just an unavoidable part of living. As we grow older, we accumulate more AGEs, and our bodies respond with the loss of elasticity and tone to skin and other tissues, decreased functional efficiency of organs, failing eyesight, declining memory, reduced ability to fight off infections, and all the other symptoms associated with aging. Some people are exposed to more AGEs than others. Diabetics are particularly troubled by these rogue molecules. The major complications associated with diabetes—failing eyesight, nerve damage, kidney failure, and heart disease—are all directly linked to AGEs.

Why are diabetics so vulnerable to these troublemakers? The answer is sugar or, more specifically, blood sugar or blood glucose. Chronically elevated blood glucose levels expose our cells and tissues to high concentrations of glucose for extended periods of time. The longer glucose is in contact with proteins, the greater the opportunity to form advanced glycation end products. High blood sugar causes accelerated AGEing.

We are not totally defenseless against AGEs, for they are so harmful that the body is equipped with some means of getting rid of them. Our white blood cells have receptors specifically designed for them. They latch on to the damaged proteins and remove them.

However, some glycated proteins, like those in collagen or nerve tissues, aren't easily removed. They tend to stick to each other and to other proteins, accumulating and causing damage to surrounding tissues. This plaque-like material becomes, more or less, a permanent fixture and a continual source of irritation. When a white blood cell encounters a glycated protein, it sets off an inflammatory reaction. The receptors for AGEs are known by the acronym RAGE, quite fitting since the reaction of white blood cells with AGEs can lead to chronic inflammation. Chronic inflammation is a characteristic of many degenerative conditions, including diabetes.

Dietary Advanced Glycation End Products

As we age, we tend to accumulate greater amounts of AGEs. Research suggests that AGEs accelerate the consequences of natural aging and associated degenerative diseases such as diabetes and dementia.[7] One study reported that in a comparison of 172 young subjects (under 45 years of age) and older subjects (over 60 years), circulating AGEs increased with age. This is expected, but the researchers also found that indicators of inflammation, oxidative stress, and insulin resistance increased with AGEs regardless of the subject's chronological age.[8] Ultimately, it was discovered that AGE levels are more important at determining functional age than chronological age. It's not how old you are but how much accumulated damage you have sustained that really determines your level of health.

Most of the AGEs in our bodies come from eating sugar and refined carbohydrates. These foods raise blood sugar, which in turn, increases the rate at which glucose in our blood attaches (glycates) to tissue proteins and fats to form AGEs. While we most often think of glucose when we talk about glycation, another sugar, fructose, undergoes glycation at about ten times the rate of glucose.

In recent years, fructose, in the form of high-fructose corn syrup, has overtaken sucrose (table sugar) as the primary sweetener in commercially prepared products. The reason for this is that fructose is nearly twice as sweet as sucrose, therefore, less of it can be used to impart the same amount of sweetness. In other words, it's cheaper and reduces manufacturing costs. High-fructose corn syrup is used in the majority of packaged foods in place of sucrose or other sugars. Look at the ingredient labels of ice cream, candy, cookies, breads, and other prepared foods. If sugar is added, it most likely is in the form of high-fructose corn syrup. Food manufacturers often simply use the term "fructose" regardless of its source.

Fructose is often recommended to diabetics and those who suffer from insulin resistance because it has less of an effect on raising blood sugar than table sugar. Ironically, however, while fructose does not affect blood sugar as dramatically as sucrose, it does greater overall damage, because it increases AGE generation and intensifies insulin resistance, making conditions worse. All sources of fructose have the same effect on the body. It does not matter if the fructose is from high-fructose corn syrup or a natural source such as agave syrup (a popular sweetener used in the health food industry). The effects are all the same.

An interesting study was conducted in Europe. Researchers took two groups of non-diabetic subjects, one vegetarian group and a group who ate a mixed diet. Diet histories were recorded, and blood tests measured AGE levels. The results were surprising. It would appear that vegetarians should have lower AGE levels because they eat a seemingly healthy diet of mostly fruits, vegetables, and grains; however, the mixed diet subjects had significantly lower AGEs compared to the vegetarians. The vegetarians ate two to three times as much fresh fruit as the mixed diet subjects, three times as much dried fruit, four times as much honey, and about the same amount of commercial sugar. Overall, their sugar intake was significantly higher, particularly in fructose. The researchers attributed the higher AGE levels in the vegetarians to their high fructose consumption.[11]

Researchers at the University of Leicester in the UK carried out a survey to evaluate the prevalence of age-related cataracts in the Asian community there. Asian and Caucasian subjects aged 40 years and over were randomly selected for the evaluation. Age-related cataracts were found to develop earlier in the Asians, and a strict vegetarian diet was found to be a significant risk factor for developing cataracts among that population. Although the reason for the higher incidence of cataracts among vegetarians was not determined, it may have been due to higher sugar intake and elevated blood levels of AGEs, which are known to cause oxidation in the lens.

AGEs accelerate the effects of aging on the eyes. High blood sugar levels cause AGEs to accumulate in the lens, retina, and throughout the central nervous system. Studies report clear associations between AGEs and development of cataracts, macular degeneration, diabetic retinopathy, as well neurodegenerative diseases of various types.[13-14] The evidence is clear: Diets high in sugar and other carbohydrates substantially increase the risks of developing age-related eye disease. In fact, it appears that keeping blood sugar within normal range is a sure way to ward off degenerative eye disease.

EXCESSIVE SUNLIGHT EXPOSURE

Sunlight damages as well as stimulates the retina, allowing us to see the world around us. Animal studies clearly show that exposure to intense bright light can damage the lens and retina. Exposure to excessive sunlight has long been believed to be associated with increased risk of cataracts and age-related macular degeneration. A landmark study in 1992, the Watermen Study, confirms this. This study involved 838 watermen (fishermen) from the Chesapeake Bay region on the Eastern coast of the United States. Over a 20-year period, those who had the greatest exposure to bright sunlight were found to be at greater risk of developing macular degeneration.[15]

In the Beaver Dam Eye Study, published in 1993, exposure to sunlight was estimated from the amount of leisure time study participants spent outdoors in summer and the use of hats with brims and sunglasses. Advanced macular degeneration was positively associated with the amount of leisure time spent outside during the summer, but wearing brimmed hats and sunglasses reduced the risk.[16] Early age-related macular degeneration was less frequent among those who used hats and sunglasses. It may be important to note that many people in this region of the United States are descendants of Nordic and Northern European immigrants and have light-colored irises; therefore, they are especially sensitive to the effects of sunlight, since eyes with light-colored irises transmit 100 times as much light as those with dark brown irises.[17]

The eyes can adapt to different light intensities in the environment. This is demonstrated in animal studies. Rats raised in dim light have higher amounts of rhodopsin (the visual pigment in the rods) than do animals raised in bright light, but the animals raised in bright light have higher retinal concentrations of protective factors; the glutathione-related antioxidant enzymes and vitamins E and C. When animals raised under the two different conditions are exposed to the same intense, constant light, those raised in dim light suffered much more severe damage to the photoreceptors. In the Beaver Dam Eye Study, subjects may have been more susceptible to the bright sunshine of spring and summer after spending the cold, dark winter indoors.

Many mechanisms may be involved in light damage to the retina, but peroxidation of polyunsaturated membrane lipids (fats) is believed to be the most significant. Lipid peroxides are toxic to the retina, and photoreceptors are rich sources of fatty acids that can be oxidized.[18] The outer segments of rods and cones have the highest concentration of polyunsaturated fatty acids in the body.

The amount of polyunsaturated fatty acids in the body tissues is reflected by the diet. A diet rich in polyunsaturated vegetable oils will enrich body tissues in these fats, thus increasing susceptibility to light-induced free-radical damage.

In light studies, most researchers have ignored the effect of diet, assuming exposure to sunlight as the only primary factor in age-related macular degeneration. However, normal sunlight is only destructive when the diet is rich in polyunsaturated oils. The eyes of people who eat less polyunsaturated vegetable oils are much more durable, even with long-term exposure to bright sunlight. If sunlight was the cause, the vast majority of our ancestors who worked outdoors all day long would have lost their eyesight due to macular degeneration and cataracts, but this was not the case. It is important to consider that they did not eat polyunsaturated vegetable oils; rather, they predominately ate saturated and monounsaturated fats like butter, cream, coconut oil, olive oil, and lard. These are traditional fats people have been eating throughout history. Only in 20th century did polyunsaturated vegetable oils become widely available and affordable.

In addition, in our modern society most people work indoors, out of the sun. We rarely go out into the sun for any period of time except on the weekends and holidays. This has, no doubt, conditioned our eyes to a dim-light environment with lower antioxidants levels. When we go outdoors, sunlight has a greater oxidizing effect.

Diet is the key to how much sunlight can harm the eyes, and it is far more important than total sun exposure. Low antioxidant intake will also increase vulnerability. Diets low in fruits and vegetables and high in processed vegetable oils, fried foods, mayonnaise made with vegetable oils, chips, cookies, and other processed foods increase susceptibility.

Most people are aware that ultraviolet (UV) light is harmful to the eyes and may lead to cataracts, macular degeneration, and other age-related eye diseases. We cannot see UV light, for it is that portion of the spectrum of invisible light below 400nm. While the primary source of UV light is the sun, other sources include welder's flash, video display terminals, fluorescent lighting, high-intensity mercury vapor lamps (for night sports and used in high-crime areas), and xenon arc lamps.

There are three types of UV light: UVA, UVB, and UVC. UVC (below 286 nm) is effectively filtered by the Earth's ozone layer. UVB (286-320 nm) is solar energy that causes sunburn and is the major risk factor for all types of skin cancers; much of it is absorbed by the cornea and does not reach the retina. UVA (320-400 nm) contributes to skin aging but can also increase risk of skin cancer, particularly when cell membranes in the skin are enriched in polyunsaturated fatty acids. The lens absorbs and filters out most of the UV light that enters the eye, to prevent it from reaching the retina. Consequently, the lens requires a high amount of antioxidants to protect it from the oxidizing effects of UV radiation.

Blue light, which is within the visible spectrum, has a wavelength between 400 and 500 nm and passes through the lens and is absorbed by the retina. It is considered less dangerous than UV light but more damaging than other wavelengths of visible light and is more likely to cause cataracts and damage the retina.

Believe it or not, people who wear corrective eyeglasses (not sunglasses) may be protected, to some extent, from the potential damaging effects of sunlight, as regular eyeglasses block out a fair amount of UV light. Ordinary glass, like the type used in windows, blocks all UVB light. Consequently, people who do not wear glasses are at greater risk for macular degeneration and cataracts. Farsighted people are more at risk than nearsighted; this is believed to be because those who are farsighted generally only wear glasses after middle age and are less protected than nearsighted people, who wear eyeglasses at all ages. If you wear contact lenses, you have no added protection, because contacts do not block any UV light.

SMOKING

Smoking has long been known to cause heart disease and cancer and increase the risk of developing diabetes. It can also greatly increase the risk of age-related eye diseases. Tobacco smoke is a major source of free radical-producing pro-oxidants that deplete the body's protective antioxidants and increases AGE formation. Blood levels of AGEs in smokers are higher than in nonsmokers.[19] Smoking leads to constriction or narrowing of the blood vessels that nourish the retina. The retina has a high rate of oxygen consumption. Anything that affects the rate of oxygen delivery to the retina has the potential to degrade retina health and negatively impact vision.

Antioxidant carotenoids, like beta-carotene and lutein, are substantially reduced in smokers. Although smokers generally have lower dietary carotenoid intake than nonsmokers, their blood carotenoid concentrations are even lower than would be predicted from the difference in diet. This suggests that the oxidant load from smoking depletes the blood of carotenoids.

Smokers also have lower blood concentrations of vitamin C. This is partly due to lower dietary intake, but even after adjusting for dietary intake they still show lower blood vitamin C concentrations.

Because of the high levels of free radicals and AGEs, the reduced delivery of oxygen, and lowered level of antioxidant vitamins, smokers are at elevated risk for all manner of degenerative eye disease. Cataracts are common among smokers, and heavy smokers (15 cigarettes or more per day) have up to three times the risk of developing cataracts. Dry eye syndrome is more than twice as common among smokers as non-smokers.

Narrowed arteries increase blood pressure in the eyes, which can lead to hemorrhaging and leaking of the tiny blood vessels feeding the retina. Damage to the retina increases susceptibility to glaucoma. In diabetics these blood vessels are already compromised, thus increasing the changes of complications associated with diabetic retinopathy.

Smokers are up to five times more likely to develop macular degeneration than nonsmokers. The risk of macular degeneration in smokers remains high even up to 15 years after quitting. Breathing secondhand smoke is almost as harmful; nonsmokers who live with smokers have almost twice the risk as those who are not regularly exposed to smoke.

DRUGS

If you looked at all of the side effects associated with many common prescription and over-the-counter medicines, you would likely be surprised to find how many adversely affect vision and eye health. It seems that if you wanted to destroy your vision, taking drugs is the quickest route to it.

Many common drugs, which we don't think twice about using, may be the underlying cause of our eye problems. Some of the most common drug-induced side effects are cataracts, dry eye, and retinal damage. For example, non-steroidal anti-inflammatory drugs (NSAIDs) such as ibuprofen (Motrin, Advil) used for pain relief can cause retinal hemorrhages (bleeding), dry eyes, and optic neuritis (inflammation of the optic nerve). Tylenol, which is not an NSAID, may be safer, but it can also affect the eyes by disturbing color vision or cause double vision.

Over-the-counter antacids like Zantac, Pepcid, and Tagamet can cause retinal hemorrhages, dry eyes, blurred vision, light sensitivity, and disturbed color vision. Some people have chronic indigestion and take these like candy, without ever realizing they are damaging brain and eye tissue. Frequent users of Zantac and other antacids have 2.5 times greater a risk of developing dementia.[20]

Antidepressants are known to cause hemorrhaging in the brain. This bleeding in the brain leads to inflammation and massive free-radical activity, causing a great deal of damage. Vision-related side effects include retinal hemorrhage, light sensitivity, dry eyes, optic neuritis, increased eye pressure, blurred vision, double vision, cataracts, eye pain, and disturbed accommodation (ability to focus). Nearly every drug designed to treat psychological disorders carries the risk of brain and eye damage. Anti-anxiety, antipsychotic, and hyperactivity medications can lead to similar range of visual side effects. Sadly, some people use these drugs every day, increasing their risk of serious and permanent harm.

Many drugs used to prevent and treat heart disease are among the worst offenders. Cholesterol-lowering drugs (statins), hypertensive (high blood pressure) drugs, and blood thinners can cause a variety of conditions, ranging from blurred vision to cataracts. Cholesterol-lowering statins are particularly troubling, as they significantly increase the risk of developing glaucoma, diabetes (insulin resistance), and dementia. Statins lower blood cholesterol by deactivating enzymes that the body uses to make cholesterol. Most of the cholesterol in the body does not come from diet; instead, it is manufactured in the liver. Cholesterol is a major component of nerve and brain tissue. It is so important to brain function that the brain does not rely solely on the cholesterol produced by the liver but also produces some on its own. Likewise, the retina contains a high percentage of cholesterol; it is vital to the function of the photoreceptors and for the transmission of visual nerve impulses to the brain. When you forcibly lower cholesterol levels with drugs, you create a cholesterol deficiency in the retina and

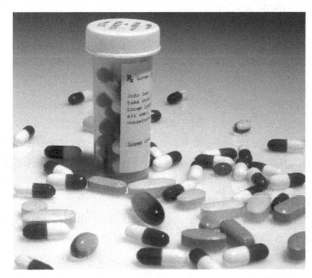

Many drugs can adversely affect eyesight and promote vision loss.

other nerve tissue, which can compromise the structure and function of the retina leading to progressive degeneration.[21]

Ironically, some medications taken for certain eye conditions lead to other eye problems and further degeneration of eye health. For example, glaucoma medications such as Betoptic and Timoptic can cause dry eyes and double vision. Allergy medications like Actifed and Benadryl are often prescribed for conjunctivitis but can dry the eyes, dilate pupils, and cause retinal hemorrhaging.

Certain antibiotics (tetracycline), antihistamines, diuretics, oral contraceptives, sleep aids (Lunesta, Ambien, Rozerem, Halcion, Sominex, and Sonata), and drugs to treat Alzheimer's (Aricept), hypothyroidism (Synthroid), COPD (Atrovent), menopause (Premarin), osteoporosis (Fosamax), migraines (Cafergot, Imitrex), and epilepsy all have the potential to adversely affect eye health.

It is not possible in the space allotted here to list all the drugs that can affect vision. In addition, new drugs are continually being developed which would be added to the list. You can find the major side effects for most any drug online by going to www.drugs.com. Not all side effects are listed. Those that simply list "vision problems" could be referring to anything from retinal hemorrhaging and glaucoma to blurred vision and dry eye. If the side effects include neurological symptoms such as hallucinations, dizziness, loss of balance, or speech difficulties or cardiovascular symptoms such as reduced blood flow or stroke, you can bet that drug will also cause damage to the brain and eyes as well. Any disturbance in the brain will affect the eyes, and if the circulatory system is adversely affected, it will influence blood circulation in the brain and eyes.

EXCITOTOXINS

To understand how degenerative eye diseases affect the eye and to evaluate possible new treatments, scientists often give lab animals a form of glutamate called N-methyl-D-aspartate (NMDA), which induces damage to the retina and optic nerve similar to that of age-related eye diseases such as glaucoma. Glutamate is an amino acid that is used as one of the primary neurotransmitters in the brain and retina. Neurotransmitters are chemicals that relay signals from one neuron to another. For example, when light triggers a chemical reaction in the photoreceptors in the retina, these signals are transmitted to the retinal ganglion cells and optic nerve by neurotransmitters. When brain cells speak to each other, they do so by sending out neurotransmitters, which are picked up by adjacent neurons.

Glutamate is normally harmless; in fact, it is necessary for cell-to-cell communication. However, in excess, it can become toxic. Glutamate is an excitatory neurotransmitter, meaning it initiates increased chemical activity. Too many can over-stimulate the neurons, exciting them into a feverish frenzy of electrical activity, exhausting the neuron's energy reserves, causing them to die. In the process, a large number of destructive free radicals are generated that promote inflammation and cellular damage. This is why it is used to study degenerative eye diseases.

Another excitatory neurotransmitter is the amino acid aspartate, which is similar to glutamate. In fact, our cells can convert aspartate into glutamate and vice versa. Aspartate and glutamate are important neurotransmitters. In fact, they are the most abundant neurotransmitters in the brain. Both are found in various levels in foods and can become potent Excitotoxins—substances that cause overstimulation leading to cellular death.

The body is capable of handling a certain amount of excess neurotransmitters, and receptors and enzymes typically keep them under control. But if the influx of neurotransmitters is greater than the body's ability to control them, brain cells can literally be stimulated to death. A few dead brain cells here and there won't be noticeable at first, but if the situation is repeated over and over again, then more and more brain cells will be killed. In time, the accumulative loss of brain and retinal cells will manifest itself as various age-related degenerative diseases.

A growing number of studies are linking glutamate and aspartate excitotoxicity to neurodegenerative diseases such as Alzheimer's, Parkinson's, ALS, Huntington's, stroke, and glaucoma.[22-30] The typical decline in vision, memory defects, mild intellectual deterioration, and loss of coordination that frequently surfaces in late middle age may be due, in part, to excessive consumption of excitotoxins.

The most frequent source of aspartate is from the artificial sweetener aspartame, commonly used to sweeten sugar-free beverages and desserts. The biggest source of glutamate is monosodium glutamate

(MSG)—a flavor enhancer. MSG is added to a large assortment of commercially packaged foods—soups, frozen dinners, pizza, gravies, sauces, chips, croutons, lunch meats, bouillon, canned tuna, and salad dressings. It is also frequently used in restaurants. It can even be purchased in the spice section of the grocery store, sold under the brand name Accent.

Processed meats such as hot dogs, ham, sausage, cold cuts, beef sticks, and jerky often have MSG added. According to the University of Illinois Eye and Ear Infirmary, one serving per day of processed meat increases risk of macular degeneration progression by 2.09 times.

The negative effects of glutamate were first observed in 1954 by a Japanese scientist who noted that direct application of glutamate to the central nervous system caused seizures. Unfortunately, this very telling report went unnoticed for several years. The toxicity of glutamate was again observed in 1957 by two ophthalmologists, D.R. Lucas and J.P. Newhouse, when it was discovered that the feeding of monosodium glutamate to newborn mice destroyed the neurons in the inner layers of the retina. Later, in 1969, neuropathologist John Olney repeated the Lucas and Newhouse experiment and discovered that the phenomenon was not restricted to the retina but occurred throughout the brain. He coined the term "excitotoxicity" to describe the neural damage that glutamate, aspartate, phenylalanine, cysteine, homocysteine, and other excitotoxins can cause.

In 1994, Russell L. Blaylock, MD, a clinical assistant professor of neurosurgery at the University of Mississippi Medical Center at the time, published a book titled *Excitotoxins: The Taste That Kills*. Both of his parents were afflicted with Parkinson's disease, which compelled him to research the disease in depth, seeking the cause and an effective treatment. His research led him to an understanding of the devastating effects of excitotoxic food additives and their influence on various forms of neurodegeneration. His book summarizes the research linking excitotoxins to neurodegenerative disease and provides details on the types of foods to avoid.

If only a few foods contained glutamate or aspartate, it wouldn't be much of a problem, as small amounts in the diet can be handled without too much worry. The problem is that the vast majority of processed, packaged, and restaurant foods contain excitotoxins. It is very difficult to find a canned, frozen, packaged, or prepared food in the grocery store that does not contain excitotoxic additives in some form.

Aspartame and MSG are the most common and the most recognizable. Due to growing public awareness of the dangers of MSG, food manufacturers often disguise this ingredient by putting it in a different form. Additives that contain MSG include hydrolyzed vegetable protein, sodium caseinate, calcium caseinate, yeast extract, autolyzed yeast, soy protein isolate, and textured protein. Of these, hydrolyzed vegetable protein is probably the worst because it also contains two other excitotoxins—aspartate and cysteine. Some food manufacturers attempt to sell the idea that the additive is all natural or safe because it is made from vegetables, but that is simply not true. Dr. Russell Blaylock says, "Experimentally, one can produce the same brain lesions using hydrolyzed vegetable protein as by using MSG or aspartate." One very ambiguous but common ingredient is "natural flavorings." Despite the claim that these are natural, this general term often includes MSG. For better eye health and overall health, get in the habit of reading the ingredients on everything you buy, and avoid all foods containing these additives or any with similar-sounding names.

Amino acids have become popular as dietary supplements, and individual purified excitotoxins are being peddled as dietary supplements labeled as L-glutamine, L-cysteine, and L-phenylalanine. You may also see them in combination with other amino acids. Despite health claims, these are nothing more than brain-destroying drugs, and it is best to avoid them all.

Some people are more sensitive to excitotoxins than others and display allergy-like reactions. This has been called "Chinese Restaurant Syndrome" because MSG is commonly used in Asian cooking. Symptoms may include headaches, nausea, diarrhea, heart palpations, dizziness, difficulty concentrating, mood swings, heartburn, skin rashes, and others. Those who are allergic to MSG are lucky, for they have learned to avoid eating foods with this additive, while the rest of us may be completely oblivious to the damage that is being done.

Those people who defend the use of MSG state that glutamate is a natural substance commonly found in many foods, that if glutamate-containing foods are not harmful, then MSG is not harmful either. Our bodies can handle natural dietary sources of glutamate that are found in meats, cheeses, vegetables, and such. This is clearly seen in those who are allergic to MSG. They can eat mushrooms, tomato sauce, red meat, and other foods high in natural glutamate without problem, but when they eat foods with added MSG, they experience immediate adverse reactions. Obviously, there is something very different between the glutamate that is found naturally in foods and the glutamate in food additives.

Protein is built from amino acids. Glutamate is one of 20 amino acids important to human health. Many plant and animal proteins in our foods contain glutamate. Glutamate in foods is always attached to other amino acids. The process of breaking proteins down into individual amino acids takes time, so the amino acids are released slowly. Blood levels of glutamate are kept within reasonable bounds that the body is capable of handling. Also, glutamate bound to other amino acids or proteins cannot pass through the blood-brain barrier, so it doesn't pose a problem. The glutamate in MSG, on the other hand, is in its free form and does not have to be broken off a protein, so you absorb a higher dose more quickly. MSG in this more purified form acts like a drug, passing through the blood-brain barrier with an immediate destructive effect.

Excess glutamate in the brain is so detrimental that it is carefully regulated by a special cleanup and recycling system. When glutamate is released by nerve cells in the normal action of relaying messages to one another, some of it tends to drift away, into the extracellular space. Special glutamate transport proteins are waiting, ready to bind to this extracellular glutamate. These proteins shuttle the excess glutamate to cells where it is stored for future use. Certain conditions, such as an influx of glutamate from the bloodstream, exposure to toxins, infection, and the release of free radicals formed by peroxidation of polyunsaturated fats, can interfere with the action of the glutamate transporters.[31-33]

High blood levels of free glutamate in the diet tend to open the blood-brain barrier, allowing more glutamate to enter the brain, along with other neurotoxins.[34] This extracellular glutamate, along with other neurotoxins interfere with glutamate transporters, trigger inflammation, and stimulate free-radical production. This excitotoxicity causes the release of intracellular glutamate stored in the brain cells. The brain is then flooded with glutamate, causing more inflammation and producing more free radicals; this, in turn, releases more glutamate. A vicious cycle continues, leading to neuron destruction.[35]

Even small concentrations of excitotoxins entering the brain can trigger this destructive cycle. Anyone who wants to avoid developing neurodegenerative diseases as they grow older, and definitely anyone who is already experiencing the effects of these disorders, should stop eating foods with excitotoxic additives immediately. Replace the processed, packaged convenience foods with fresh, natural foods, and make more meals from scratch rather than using packaged ingredients. When you go out to eat, it is difficult to avoid all possible sources of MSG, but you can reduce a lot if you tell them that you do not want MSG in your food. Often they can accommodate you, but sometimes the packaged foods they use already have the ingredient in it. Choose items on the menu that are MSG free.

Likewise, you should avoid all foods containing aspartame. Brand names for aspartame include NutraSweet, Equal, Sugar Twin, and AminoSweet. Also, as a reminder, you should get into the habit of reading all ingredient labels before purchasing any packaged or bottled food.

5

Blood Sugar and Insulin Resistance

DIABETES AND NEURODEGENERATION

Diabetes is a major cause of disability leading to blindness, lower-limb amputation, kidney disease, and nerve damage. According to the American Academy of Ophthalmology, people with diabetes are 25 times more likely to become blind than people without diabetes. Currently, 29 million Americans, 9.3 percent of the U.S. population, have diabetes, and over 8 million are living with diabetes without even being aware of it. More than 26 percent of all adults age 65 and older have diabetes. That's one out of every four older adults! But it's not just an old-age disease; over 200,000 people under the age of 20 have been diagnosed with the disease as well. Among all age groups, over 1.7 million new cases are diagnosed each year. There are many more people, 86 million, age 20 years and over, who are pre-diabetic. All of these people are at risk of developing visual problems at some point in their lives. The younger the patient is at the time of diabetes diagnosis, the greater the risk. Diabetes is not just an American problem, the rate of diabetes is increasing rapidly worldwide.

Diabetes occurs as a result of the body's inability to properly regulate blood sugar. When we eat, much of the food is converted into glucose, or blood sugar, and sent into the bloodstream. When blood sugar levels rise too high, the body is thrown into a panic, metabolically speaking. The pancreas releases insulin into the bloodstream to shuttle glucose into the cells and lower blood sugar levels; however, if blood sugar is not normalized in a reasonable amount of time, cells and tissues become damaged. This is what happens in people with diabetes.

There are different types of diabetes. The most common are type 1 and type 2. Type 1 occurs when the pancreas stops producing insulin or produces too little to effectively reduce blood glucose. Type 1 diabetes is typically diagnosed in early childhood and is also known as juvenile-onset diabetes or insulin-dependent diabetes mellitus. Type 1 diabetics require a lifetime of regular insulin injections to keep blood sugar in balance. This form of diabetes can develop in older individuals due to dysfunction of the pancreas by alcohol abuse or disease, but it comprises less than 10 percent of all cases of diabetes.

In type 2 diabetics, the pancreas may be capable of producing a normal amount of insulin, but the cells of the body have become unresponsive or resistant to its action. Thus, a larger amount of insulin is needed to remove glucose from the bloodstream and put it in the cells. This condition is known as insulin resistance. This is by far the most common form of diabetes. About 90 percent of diabetics are of this type. Type 2 diabetes typically occurs in adulthood. Early in the course of the disease the pancreas is usually capable of producing the large amounts of insulin needed to overcome the insulin resistance of the cells, but over time, the high demand for insulin takes its toll on the pancreas, and insulin production begins to decline. More than half of those with type 2 diabetes eventually require insulin shots to control their blood sugar levels as they age. Type 2 diabetes is usually controlled with diet, weight management, exercise, and medication.

A third form of diabetes has recently been recognized. This newly discovered type of diabetes links insulin resistance with neurodegeneration, most specifically with Alzheimer's disease. Alzheimer's is essentially diabetes, or insulin resistance, of the brain and is referred to as type 3 diabetes.[1] The fact that Alzheimer's is recognized as a form of diabetes is not as strange as it might sound, for diabetes has long been known to adversely affect nerve tissue throughout the body, including the brain.

Insulin resistance can have an adverse effect on virtually every organ and system in the body. Chronic insulin resistance causes nerve damage, a condition known as diabetic neuropathy, and is the most common serious complication of diabetes. About 60 to 70 percent of people with diabetes have some form of neuropathy. Symptoms include pain, tingling, or numbness in the hands, arms, feet, and legs. The legs and feet are the most commonly affected, but nerve damage can develop throughout the body.

Population-based studies have shown that those with type 2 diabetes have an increased risk of cognitive impairment, dementia, and neurodegeneration.[2] Diabetics have almost twice the risk of developing Alzheimer's disease as the general population.[3] The younger a person is when he or she develops insulin resistance, the greater the risk. If diabetes occurs before the age of 65, it is associated with a 125 percent increased risk of eventually developing Alzheimer's disease.[4] Insulin resistance does not have to be in the diabetes range to increase the risk of Alzheimer's, even pre-diabetics are in danger of developing the disease.

Any disturbance in normal insulin function can dramatically affect energy metabolism and, consequently, brain function. All major neurodegenerative diseases, including vascular dementia, Parkinson's disease, Huntington's disease, MS, and ALS, exhibit features suggesting insulin resistance as either an important underlying factor or a contributor to the initiation and progression of these diseases.[5-7] In that sense, they could all be viewed as various manifestations of type 3 diabetes.

For example, research is just now beginning to uncover the relationships between Parkinson's disease and insulin resistance.[8] Insulin resistance has been reported in up to 80 percent of Parkinson's disease patients. Dysfunction of insulin metabolism in the brain is known to precede the death of the dopamine-producing neurons in the development of Parkinson's disease.[9] Insulin resistance also exacerbates the severity of the symptoms and reduces the therapeutic efficacy of medications used to treat the disease.[10] In one of the largest studies of this kind to date, researchers followed a group of more than 50,000 men and women over a period of 18 years. The researchers found that those people who had type 2 diabetes at the start of the study were 83 percent more likely to be diagnosed with Parkinson's disease later in life than non-diabetics.[11] If the study had been carried on over a longer period of time, there is no doubt there would have been an even greater correlation, since the risk of Parkinson's increases with age.

Likewise, studies show that insulin resistance greatly increases the risk of developing cataracts, glaucoma, and macular edema (fluid buildup behind the macula). It accelerates vision loss in macular degeneration and, of course, is the cause of diabetic retinopathy one of the major complications resulting from diabetes.[12-14]

GLUCOSE POWERS OUR CELLS

The cells in the brain and eyes, as well as every other organ in the body, require energy in order to perform their various functions. We derive energy from the three major nutrients: carbohydrate, protein, and fat. While protein and fat can produce energy when necessary, their primary function in the human body is to provide the basic building blocks for tissues, hormones, enzymes, and other structures. The primary purpose of carbohydrate, on the other hand, is to produce energy. It is the body's preferred choice for fuel. Typically, 55 to 60 percent of our energy needs are supplied by carbohydrate with the remainder coming from protein and fat.

Plants are made predominantly of carbohydrates. Milk is the only animal-derived food that contains any significant amount of carbohydrate. Carbohydrates are constructed of sugar; thus in essence, sugar molecules provide the basic building blocks for all plants. The vegetables in your refrigerator are composed almost entirely of sugar and water.

There are three basic types of sugar molecules that are important in our diet—glucose, fructose, and galactose. All the carbohydrates in our diet consist of some combination of these three. Simple carbohydrates consist of only one or two units of sugar. For example, table sugar, or sucrose, is a mixture of glucose and fructose. One molecule of sucrose consists of one molecule of glucose and one of fructose. Milk sugar, or lactose, consists of one molecule of glucose and one of galactose. Complex carbohydrates are composed of many sugar molecules linked together by chemical bonds. Starch, for example, consists of long chains of glucose. Glucose is by far the most abundant sugar molecule in plant foods.

When you eat a slice of bread, you are eating mostly glucose in the form of starch. Along with the starch, you get some water, fiber (which is also a type of carbohydrate), vitamins, and minerals. The same is true when you eat an apple, a carrot, corn, potatoes, or any other plant-derived food.

When food containing carbohydrate is consumed, digestive enzymes break the bonds between the sugar molecules, releasing the individual glucose, fructose, and galactose molecules. These sugars are then transported to the bloodstream. From there, glucose is delivered throughout the body to supply the fuel needed by the cells. Fructose and galactose, in their original form, cannot be used by the cells to produce energy. They are taken up by the liver, converted into glucose, then released back into the bloodstream. Foods high in glucose produce a rapid rise in blood sugar concentration. Fructose and galactose increase blood sugar as well, but not as rapidly since they must pass through the liver first.

Dietary fiber is also a carbohydrate, but the human body does not produce the enzymes necessary to break the chemical bonds that hold these sugars together. Therefore, fiber passes through the digestive tract and out of the body mostly intact. Since fiber releases little or no sugar, it does not raise blood sugar levels.

Most cells cannot store glucose. Rather, they take from the bloodstream and use what is necessary for their immediate needs. The liver and muscle cells are exceptions; they have the ability to store a small amount of glucose in the form of glycogen for later use. Most of the excess sugar is converted into fat and stored in fat cells.

If food is not consumed for a period of time and the stored glucose becomes depleted, the body begins to metabolize fat and protein to meet its energy needs. Fat serves as the primary alternative source of energy when blood glucose levels decline. To a limited extent, protein can be converted into glucose, fat however, cannot. It is released as individual fat molecules known as fatty acids. Some of these fatty acids are converted into molecular units called ketone bodies or ketones. Fatty acids and ketones can be used by the cells in place of glucose to supply energy needs.

THE ROLE OF INSULIN

As glucose circulates throughout the body, it is picked up by the cells and transformed into energy. The cells, however, cannot absorb glucose by themselves and require the help of the hormone insulin. Insulin unlocks the door on the cell membrane, allowing glucose to enter; without insulin, glucose cannot enter the cells. Your blood could be saturated with glucose, but if insulin was not present, glucose could not pass though the cell membrane, and the cells would "starve" and die.

Every cell in your body requires a continuous supply of fuel to function normally. Just like us, if we don't get enough food at regular intervals, our health fails and we die. Likewise, if the cells don't get enough glucose on a continual basis, they degenerate and die.

But an overabundance of glucose is not good either. Too much glucose is toxic. In order to avoid the dire consequences of too little or too much glucose, the body carefully maintains a narrow range of glucose levels in the blood.

Blood sugar levels naturally fluctuate slightly throughout the day. Whenever we eat, our blood sugar levels increase. Between meals or during times of heavy physical activity, as the body's demand for energy increases, blood sugar levels decline. Glucose, stored in the liver in the form of glycogen, is released to maintain blood sugar levels. As long as the body is capable of compensating for upward and downward spikes in blood sugar, balance is quickly reestablished and maintained.

What we eat profoundly affects the workings of this system. Meals high in carbohydrates—especially those that contain a significant amount of simple carbohydrates and lack fiber, fat, and protein—can cause blood glucose levels to rise very rapidly. Refined starches such as white flour have been stripped of most of their fiber and bran and tend to act like sugar, spiking blood glucose levels as well.

Fiber, protein, and especially fat, slows digestion and absorption of carbohydrates, so glucose trickles gradually into the bloodstream, providing a steady, ongoing supply. The larger the quantity of simple, refined carbohydrates in meals, the greater the spike in blood sugar and the greater the strain placed on the body and especially the pancreas, which produces insulin.

If a high-carb meal is eaten every four or five hours, along with one or two high-carb snacks, blood glucose and insulin levels are going to be raised continually for a substantial part of the day. When cells are continuously exposed to high insulin levels, they begin to lose their sensitivity to the hormone. It is something like walking into a room with a bad odor. When you first enter the room the smell can be overpowering, but if you have to stay in the room for any length of

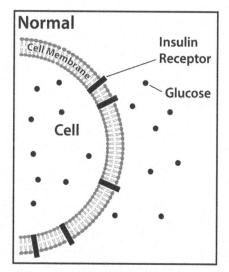
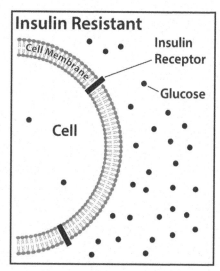

Fewer insulin receptors are available in a state of insulin resistance, resulting in a reduction of glucose entering the cells and an increase in blood glucose levels.

time, the smell receptors in your nose become desensitized and you will not notice the odor any longer. The smell is still there, but your ability to detect it declines. If you leave the room for a while and your sense of smell became resensitized, as soon as you walked back into the room you would again notice the odor. Our bodies react to insulin in somewhat the same way. Chronic exposure to high insulin levels desensitizes the cells, and they become unresponsive or resistant to the action of insulin. This is referred to as insulin resistance. In order to move glucose into the cells, a higher-than-normal concentration of insulin is necessary, but this puts more stress on the pancreas to produce the hormone in greater quantities. For this reason, diet has a direct affect on the development of insulin resistance and, consequently, diabetes and all the complications associated with it.

INSULIN RESISTANCE

If you are an average, non-diabetic individual, when you wake up in the morning, your blood contains between 65 and 100 mg/dl (3.6 and 5.5 mmol/l) of glucose. This is known as the fasting blood glucose concentration. Fasting blood sugar measurements are taken after a person has not eaten for at least eight hours. The ideal fasting blood sugar range is between 75 to 90 mg/dl (4.2 to 5.0 mmol/l).

When you don't eat, and as your cells continue to draw glucose out of the blood, your glucose level gradually falls. Normally, after eating a meal, your blood sugar should not rise to more than 139 mg/dl (7.7 mmol/l). This is called postprandial glucose level. Elevated fasting and postprandial glucose levels indicate insulin resistance.

Diabetes is diagnosed when fasting blood sugar is 126 mg/dl (7.0 mmol/l) or higher. People with fasting blood sugar levels between 101 and 125 mg/dl (5.6 and 6.9 mmol/l) are considered to be in the early stages of diabetes, often referred to as "pre-diabetes." Fasting blood sugar levels over 90 mg/dl (5.0 mmol/l) indicate the beginning stages of insulin resistance. As insulin resistance increases, so do blood sugar levels. The higher your blood sugar is, the more insulin resistant you are, and the greater your risk of neurodegeneration and eye damage.

The level at which a person is considered to have full-blown diabetes is more or less arbitrary. For many years, a fasting blood sugar reading of 140 mg/dl (7.8 mmol/l) defined diabetes. In 1997, however, The American Diabetes Association lowered the definition to 126 mg/dl (7.0 mmol.l). Does this mean that if you have fasting blood sugar of 125 mg/dl (6.9 mmol/l), you are not diabetic and have none of the associated health risks? Not hardly, because in reality, the 126 mg/dl (7.0 mmol/l) is just as arbitrary as 140 mg/dl (7.8 mmol/l). Insulin resistance is typically present in anyone who has a fasting blood sugar level over 90 mg/dl (5.0 mmol/l). Although levels up to 100 mg/dl (5.5 mmol/l) are generally considered normal, they are only viewed as such because so many people fit into this category; these levels are not, in fact, normal for a "healthy" individual. Insulin resistance is not healthy, even if the condition is relatively mild. About 80 percent of the population is insulin resistant to some degree, meaning fasting blood sugar levels above 90 mg/dl (5.0 mmol/l). Consequently, many people are at increased risk of experiencing health problems associated with this condition, including visual problems. You don't need to be diagnosed with diabetes in order to develop glaucoma or cataracts— even pre-diabetics are at increased risk.

Diabetes has reached epidemic proportions. According to the Mayo Clinic, diabetes has doubled in the United States over the past 15 years. Worldwide, diabetes has increased from 30 million to 230 million cases over the past two decades, nearly an eightfold increase! This has been documented in the Japanese, Israelis, Africans, Native Americans, Eskimos, Polynesians, Micronesians, and others.[15] This frightening and phenomenal increase is believed to be due to the increased consumption of refined grains and sugars. Animal studies have shown that diets very high in sugar cause insulin resistance and diabetes, so it is reasonable to conclude that the change in dietary habits in humans over the past several decades is at the core of our current diabetes epidemic.

Some people are more susceptible to diabetes or insulin resistance than others, and this susceptibility can be due to the behaviors of the parents, albeit this is not technically genetic. Children of diabetic parents are at higher risk of developing insulin resistance and becoming diabetic themselves. If just one parent is insulin resistant, even if it is not severe enough to be diagnosed as full-fledged diabetes, children are at greater risk of developing insulin resistance. Mothers who develop gestational diabetes predispose their children to develop insulin resistance later in life. This is why diabetes sometimes seems to run in families. Susceptibility does not come from poor genes; rather, it is a result of nutritional deficiencies. In other words, it is passed on to future generations as a consequence of a poor diet. To make matters worse, poor eating habits are taught to children, who pass it down to their own offspring, resulting in a continuous cycle of poor health. Consequently, people are developing diabetes at increasingly earlier ages.

In 1997, the United States government recommended that all adults be tested for diabetes by the time they reach age 45, before diabetic complications can progress and become difficult to treat. Testing people at 45 may be too late. The average age at which diabetes is diagnosed now has decreased to 37. Researchers from the Centers for Disease Control and Prevention (CDC) now recommend that people should be tested for type 2 diabetes at age 25.

Inheriting a susceptibility for insulin resistance or diabetes doesn't guarantee that these conditions will manifest, as they only develop under the right conditions. In this case, the right conditions are consuming high amounts of carbohydrate, especially refined carbohydrates and sweets. The good news is that a susceptible person can live a long healthy life, without the slightest trouble with insulin resistance, as long as he or she eats a healthy diet.

BLOOD SUGAR AND VISION LOSS

Diabetics often experience blurred vision, since high blood sugar causes changes in the retina. Blurred vision may, in fact, be the first sign of diabetes. One of the major complications of insulin resistance is diabetic retinopathy, which involves the slow degeneration of the retina. There is no question that insulin resistance threatens vision; patients with diabetes develop cataracts at an earlier age and are nearly twice as likely to develop glaucoma as compared to non-diabetics. More than half those with diabetes have a least some degree of retinopathy.

Insulin resistance in the body, at any level, promotes insulin resistance in the brain. This affects the blood-brain barrier, making it insulin resistant, thus impeding the flow of insulin into the brain. With less insulin available, the cells in the brain and eyes cannot effectively absorb glucose. As a result, these cells begin to starve, degenerate, and die. In addition, glucose levels build up in the brain, accelerating AGE formation, which promotes oxidative stress and inflammation; all of this wreaks havoc on the tissues in the central nervous system. It is no wonder that insulin resistance is associated with all major neurodegenerative disorders, including eye disease and visual complications.

If you have problems with cataracts, glaucoma, macular degeneration, or any other age-related eye disorder, you are most likely insulin resistant, at least to some degree. As one example, the higher a person's blood sugar is, the greater the risk of cataract. Researchers at Yale University studied the effects of three diets—high-carb, high-protein, and high-fat—on the incidence of cataracts in diabetic rats. As expected, blood sugar levels were highest on the high-carb diet and lowest on the high-fat diet. Development of cataracts was highest in the rats fed a high-carb diet; a lesser incidence was observed in the high-protein fed animals, while no cataracts developed in rats fed a high-fat diet.[16] Although all the rats in this study were diabetic, their diets—not the disease—determined the level of cataracts they developed. The higher the blood sugar levels, the greater the incidence of cataracts. When blood sugar was controlled by a high-fat, low-carb diet, no cataracts developed. This effect is similar in humans, as better blood sugar control has shown similar results.[17]

Whether you are diabetic or not, eating a high-carb diet will elevate blood sugar and keep it elevated for extended periods of time, increasing your risk of damage to the brain and eyes. Scientists working for the U.S. Agricultural Research Service tracked 471 middle-aged women over a 14-year period. The researchers found that the women with an average daily carbohydrate intake between 200 and 268 grams, typical for most women of normal weight, were 2.5 times more likely to get cataracts than those who consumed between 101 and 185 grams per day. Although the consumption of 101 to 185 grams per day is lower than average, it is not considered low-carb. Low-carb diets generally include no more than 100 grams of carbohydrate a day and very low-carb diets restrict it to less than 25 grams. We can conclude from this research that even a modest reduction in carbohydrate intake, and the corresponding drop in blood sugar levels, can significantly reduce risk of cataracts.[18]

Fasting blood sugar measures the glucose levels at the time of testing. Another way of measuring blood sugar is the A1C test, which gives an average over the previous three-months. Researchers at the University of Oxford found that type 2 diabetics who lower their A1C level by just 1 percent can reduce their risk of cataracts by 19 percent.[19] It appears that even a small decrease in average blood sugar can make a big impact on eye health.

The Diabetes Control and Complications Trial (DCCT) showed that better control of blood sugar levels also substantially slows the onset and progression of retinopathy.[20] Diabetics who kept their blood sugar levels as close to normal as possible also had much less kidney and nerve disease. Better control also reduces the need for sight-saving laser surgery.

Blood sugar levels increase the risk and progression of macular degeneration. According to the University of Illinois Eye and Ear Infirmary, one serving per day of processed baked goods (e.g., a slice of bread, a bagel, pie, cake, or cookie) increases risk of macular degeneration progression by 2.42 times. On the flipside, simply reducing your intake of high-carb foods by one serving per day can reduce your risk by 2.42 times.

Elevated blood sugar levels, even those considered generally being within typical or average range, accelerates brain aging and degeneration.[21] Any chronic elevation of blood sugar is harmful to the brain and eyes, so even those with so-called normal fasting glucose levels may be at increased risk. If your fasting glucose levels are above 90 mg/dl, you are at risk, and the higher the level, the greater that risk.

The bitter truth is that you may be at risk of developing an age-related eye disease, even if you have no known visual difficulties; we are all at risk. Degenerative diseases of the brain and eyes don't appear overnight; rather, they take years, even decades to develop. Glucose metabolism becomes abnormal one to two decades before type 2 diabetes is diagnosed.[22] In the meantime, the damage done can be extensive, far before any symptoms become noticeable. For example, as much as 80 percent of tissues involved may be damaged before a person can be diagnosed with Alzheimer's or Parkinson's disease, and a substantial degree of peripheral vision may be lost due to glaucoma before anything is noticed. Since no pain or sudden changes in vision are noticed, the gradual loss of sight is not easily recognized until substantial damaged has occurred. Even though you may not notice any serious problem with your vision now, it is possible that your eyes have already experienced some degree of abnormal degeneration. If you wait until symptoms become noticeable, it may be to too late to fully correct the problem.

Unlike the brain, which is inaccessible and not easily observed, the eyes can be carefully examined without too much difficulty. Your eye doctor can tell if you are developing a problem, oftentimes before it is too late. For this reason, it is a good idea to have your eyes examined periodically. Also, you should have your fasting blood glucose levels checked every few years. If your blood sugar is high, take steps now to correct the problem and you will greatly reduce your risk of experiencing vision loss later on.

6

What You Should Know About Fats and Oils

FATTY ACIDS AND TRIGLYCERIDES

The type of fats in your diet can have a very pronounced affect on your overall health as well as your visual health. For this reason, it is important that you understand which fats promote good vision and which may be harmful.

The words "fat" and "oil" are often used interchangeably. While there is no real difference, fats are generally solid at room temperature, while oils are liquid. Lard, for example, is referred to as a fat, while liquid corn oil would be called an oil.

Fats and oils are composed of fat molecules known as fatty acids. Fatty acids can be classified into three categories, depending on their degree of saturation: saturated, monounsaturated, and polyunsaturated. You may be familiar with these terms, but what constitutes an unsaturated fat, and what are the saturated ones saturated with?

Fatty acids consist almost entirely of two elements: carbon (C) and hydrogen (H). The carbon atoms are hooked together like links in a long chain. Attached to each carbon atom are two hydrogen atoms. In a saturated fatty acid, each carbon atom is attached to a pair of hydrogen atoms. In other words, it is saturated with as many hydrogen atoms as it can possibly hold. Hydrogen atoms are always attached in pairs. If one pair of hydrogen atoms is missing, this creates a monounsaturated fatty acid; "mono" indicates one pair of hydrogen atoms is missing, while "unsaturated" indicates that the fatty acid is not fully saturated with hydrogen atoms. If two, three, or more pairs

```
    H H H H H  H H  H H  H H H H H H H H O
    | | | | |  | |  | |  | | | | | | | | ‖
H–C–C–C–C–C–C–C–C–C–C–C–C–C–C–C–C–C–C–O–H
    | | | | |  | |  | |  | | | | | | | |
    H H H H H H H H H H H H H H H H H
```

An 18 carbon chain saturated fatty acid.

```
    H H H H H H H H         H H H H H H H H O
    | | | | | | | |         | | | | | | | | ‖
H–C–C–C–C–C–C–C–C–C=C–C–C–C–C–C–C–C–C–O–H
    | | | | | | | |         | | | | | | | |
    H H H H H H H H H H H H H H H H H
```

An 18 carbon chain monounsaturated fatty acid.

```
    H H H H H         H         H H H H H H H H O
    | | | | |         |         | | | | | | | | ‖
H–C–C–C–C–C–C=C–C–C=C–C–C–C–C–C–C–C–C–O–H
    | | | | | | | |           | | | | | | | |
    H H H H H H H H H H H H H H H H H
```

An 18 carbon chain polyunsaturated fatty acid.

of hydrogen atoms are missing, this is a polyunsaturated fatty acid, as "poly" refers to more than one.

The fatty acids in the oil you pour on your salad for dinner and in the meat and vegetables you eat—in fact, even the fat in your own body—are in the form of triglycerides. A triglyceride is nothing more than three fatty acids joined together by a glycerol molecule. Thus, we have saturated triglycerides, monounsaturated triglycerides, or polyunsaturated triglycerides.

All vegetable oils and animal fats contain a mixture of saturated, monounsaturated, and polyunsaturated fatty acids. To say that any particular oil is saturated or monounsaturated is a gross oversimplification. No oil is purely saturated or polyunsaturated. Olive oil is often called a "monounsaturated" oil because it is *predominantly* monounsaturated, but like all vegetable oils, it also contains some polyunsaturated and saturated fatty acids as well.

Generally, animal fats contain the highest amount of saturated fatty acids, and vegetable oils contain the highest amount of polyunsaturated fatty acids. Palm and coconut oils are exceptions; although they are vegetable oils, they contain a high amount of saturated fat.

MEDIUM CHAIN TRIGLYCERIDES

The different types of fatty acids can also be classified into three major categories, depending on their size or, more precisely, the length of their carbon chains: long chain fatty acids (13 to 22 carbons), medium chain fatty acids (6 to 12 carbons), and short chain fatty acids (3 to 5 carbons). When a triglyceride is composed of three medium chain fatty acids, it is referred to as a medium chain triglyceride (MCT), likewise with long chain triglycerides (LCT) and short chain triglycerides (SCT).

LCTs are by far the most plentiful in our diet, comprising 97 percent of the triglycerides we consume. MCTs make up most of the remaining 3 percent, and SCTs are very scarce. Fatty acids with chain lengths of 12 carbons or less are metabolized differently than those containing 14 or more.

Most fats and oils are composed of 100 percent LCTs. There are very few dietary sources of MCTs. By far the richest natural source of MCTs is coconut oil, which consists of 63 percent medium chain triglycerides. The next largest source of MCTs is palm kernel oil, at 53 percent. Butter is a distant third, containing only 12 percent medium and short chain fatty acids. Milk from all species of mammals, contains MCTs. MCTs are essential for brain development in infants, supplying 25 percent of the brain's energy needs.

POLYUNSATURATED FATS
The Essential Fatty Acids

Polyunsaturated fats are found most abundantly in plants. Vegetable oils—such as soybean, safflower, sunflower, cottonseed, corn, and flaxseed oil—are composed predominantly of polyunsaturated fatty acids; therefore, these are commonly referred to as polyunsaturated oils.

Some fatty acids are classified as essential. This means our bodies cannot make them from other nutrients, so we must have them in our diet in order to achieve and maintain good health. Our bodies can manufacture saturated and monounsaturated fats from other foods. However, we do not have the ability to manufacture polyunsaturated fats. Therefore, it is essential that they be included in our diet.

When we talk about saturated, monounsaturated, or poly-unsaturated fats, we are not referring to just three types of fatty acids, but three families of fatty acids. There are many different types of saturated fatty acids, as well as many different monounsaturated and polyunsaturated fatty acids. Two families of polyunsaturated fatty acids are important to human health: omega-6 and omega-3 polyunsaturated fatty acids, and there are several varieties of each of these. Two, linoleic acid and alpha-linolenic acid, are considered essential because the body can use these to make all the rest. These are the essential fatty acids (EFAs) nutritionists often talk about. Linoleic acid belongs to the omega-6 family, and alpha-linolenic acid belongs to the omega-3 family.

Theoretically, if you eat an adequate source of linoleic acid, the body can make all the other omega-6 fatty acids it needs. Likewise, if you have an adequate source of alpha-linolenic acid, it can make all the other omega-3 fatty acids. Flaxseed oil is a rich source of alpha-linolenic acid.

Nutritional studies indicate that we need about 3 percent of our total calories to come from EFAs. In a typical 2,000 calorie diet, this is equivalent to about 7 grams, which isn't very much; a teaspoon is 5 grams. So 1½ teaspoons or ½ tablespoon of EFAs will amply supply minimum daily needs.

Since these fatty acids are considered "essential," people often get the impression that they possess special health properties and that the more they eat the better. But this is not necessarily the case. While we must have some in our diet, too much can be detrimental. Researchers have found that the consumption of polyunsaturated oil, most notably omega-6 oils, exceeding just 10 percent of total calories can lead to blood disorders, cancer, liver damage, and vitamin deficiencies.[1]

Lipid Peroxidation

One of the reasons polyunsaturated fats have the potential to cause health problems is because they are highly vulnerable to oxidation. When polyunsaturated fats oxidize, they become toxic. Oxidized fats are rancid fats. Free radicals are a product of oxidation.

When oxygen reacts normally with a compound, the compound becomes "oxidized." This process is called oxidation. Polyunsaturated fats readily oxidize via a process biochemists call lipid peroxidation. "Lipid" is the term biochemists use to designate fat or oil, and "peroxidation" signifies an oxidation process involving unsaturated fats that produce peroxide free radicals.

When polyunsaturated oils are exposed to heat, light, or oxygen, they spontaneously oxidize and form destructive free radicals. Once they are formed, free radicals can attack unsaturated fats and proteins, causing them to become oxidized and generate more free radicals. It is a self-perpetuating process.

Liquid vegetable oils can be deceiving because they look and taste harmless, even after they become rancid. The oil may not smell bad and may look as fresh as the day you bought it, yet be teaming with free radical terrorists.

When oil is extracted from seeds, the oxidation process is set in motion. The more the oil is exposed to heat, light, and oxygen, the more oxidized it becomes. By the time the oil is processed and bottled, it has already become oxidized to some extent. As it sits in the warehouse, the back of a truck, the grocery store, and your kitchen cabinet, it continues to oxidize. When you buy vegetable oil from the store, it has already gone rancid to some degree. In one study, various oils obtained off the shelf from local stores were tested for oxidation of the polyunsaturated fatty acids.[2] The researchers found that oxidation was already present in every sample tested. When you use these oils in cooking, oxidation is greatly accelerated. This is why you should never cook foods using any polyunsaturated oil. Oils that typically contain a high percentage of polyunsaturated fatty acids include: soybean, corn, safflower, sunflower, cottonseed, and peanut.

Oxidation occurs inside our bodies as well. Our only defense against free radicals is antioxidants, which stop the chain reactions that create new free radicals. If we consume too much processed vegetable oil, the free radicals they create deplete antioxidant nutrients such as vitamins A, C, and E, as well as zinc and selenium and can actually cause nutrient deficiencies.

Polyunsaturated fatty acids are found in all of our cells to one degree or another. A polyunsaturated fatty acid in a cell membrane attacked by a free radical will oxidize and become a free radical itself, then attack a neighboring polyunsaturated molecule, likely in the same cell. This destructive chain reaction continues until the cell is severely crippled or utterly destroyed. Random free-radical reactions occur throughout the body day after day, year after year, and this takes a major toll on your health.

Several studies have shown a relationship between processed vegetable oil consumption and damage to the central nervous system. In one study, for example, the effect of dietary oils on the mental ability of rats was determined by analyzing the animal's maze-learning capabilities. Various oils were added to the rats' food. The study commenced after rats had aged considerably, having allowed enough time for the effects of the oils to become measurable. Rats were then tested, and the number of their maze errors was recorded. The animals that performed the best and retained their mental capacities the longest were those that had been fed saturated fats. Those given polyunsaturated oils lost their mental abilities more quickly.[3]

The retina has a high content of polyunsaturated fatty acids and the highest oxygen uptake and glucose oxidation relative to any other tissue in the human body. It is also exposed to oxidizing radiation from sunlight. This renders the retina and surrounding tissues more susceptible to oxidative stress than any tissue in the body.[4-7] Lipid peroxidation has been identified as the major cause of retinal degeneration. A number of studies suggest that the primary culprit behind macular degeneration is the excessive consumption of unsaturated vegetables oils.[8-10] There is a considerable amount peroxidation of the unsaturated fatty acids in cell membranes within the lens of the eye, suggesting that a diet high in polyunsaturated fat contributes to cataracts.[11] Oxidative stress is also a major contributing factor to diabetic retinopathy; in fact, it plays an integral role in all major degenerative eye disorders.[12] Oxidative stress is considered a strong stimulus for the release of cytokines that activate inflammation.

In contrast, saturated fats are very resistant to oxidation. They do not form destructive free radicals. On the contrary, they act more like protective antioxidants because they prevent oxidation and the formation of free radicals. A diet high in protective saturated fats can help prevent lipid peroxidation.

Polyunsaturated fatty acids are very easily oxidized. Saturated fatty acids are very resistant to oxidization. Monounsaturated fatty acids are in between. They are more stable than polyunsaturated fatty acids but less stable than saturated fatty acids.

Replacing polyunsaturated fats with saturated and monounsaturated fats in the diet can help reduce the risks associated with free radicals. Also, eating a diet rich in antioxidant nutrients such as vitamin E and beta-carotene will help protect the polyunsaturated fatty acids in your body from oxidation.

Heat-Damaged Vegetable Oils

Most cooks recommend polyunsaturated vegetable oils in cooking and food preparation as a "healthy" alternative to saturated fats. Ironically, these unsaturated vegetable oils, when used in cooking, form a variety of toxic compounds that are far more damaging to health than any saturated fat could possibly be. Polyunsaturated vegetable oils are the least suitable for cooking.[14]

When vegetable oils are heated, these unstable polyunsaturated fatty acids are easily transformed into harmful compounds, including a particularly insidious one known as 4-hydroxy-trans-2-nonenal (4-HNE). When you cook with polyunsaturated oils, your food is littered with these toxic substances.

Even heating these oils at low temperatures causes damage to the delicate chemical structure of polyunsaturated fatty acids. Cooking foods at high temperatures accelerates oxidation and harmful chemical reactions. Numerous studies, in some cases published as early as the 1930s, have reported the toxic effects of consuming heated vegetable oils.[2]

Over the past 20 years, an increasing number of studies have found links between 4-HNE and increased risk for heart disease, stroke, Parkinson's disease, Alzheimer's disease, Huntington's disease, liver problems, osteoarthritis, and cancer. Every time you use unsaturated vegetable oils for cooking or baking, you are creating 4-HNE.

One of the conditions linked to 4-HNE in heated vegetable oils is heart disease. This may come as a surprise to most people because polyunsaturated vegetable oils are supposed to be heart friendly, yet recent studies show a clear link between 4-HNE and heart disease.[15-17] Studies also show that 4-HNE levels are high in the diseased regions of the brain in Alzheimer's patients.[18-19]

Studies show that diets containing heat-treated liquid vegetable oils produce more atherosclerosis than those containing unheated vegetable oil.[20] Any unsaturated vegetable oil can become toxic when heated, and even a small amount, especially if eaten frequently over time, will negatively affect your health. Oxidized oils have been found to induce damage to blood vessel walls and cause numerous organ lesions in animals.

The oils that are most vulnerable to the damage caused by heating are those that contain the highest amount of polyunsaturated fatty acids. Monounsaturated fatty acids are chemically more stable and can withstand higher temperatures, but they, too, can oxidize and form toxic byproducts if heated to high temperatures. Saturated fatty acids are very heat-stable and can withstand relatively high temperatures without oxidation. Therefore, saturated fats are the safest for day-to-day cooking and baking.

We need some polyunsaturated fats in our diet, but if all commercial polyunsaturated vegetable oils are rancid to some degree before we even purchase them, and if they become more harmful to health when used in cooking, how are we to obtain our daily requirement of essential fatty acids? The answer is simple. You can get your EFA requirement just as your ancestors did—from foods! You do not need to eat processed vegetable oils to satisfy your daily EFA requirements. You can get all your EFAs from food. This is by far the best way to get them because while they are still packaged in their original cellular containers, they are shielded from the damaging effects of oxygen and protected by naturally occurring antioxidants to keep them fresh.

Omega-6 essential polyunsaturated fatty acids are found in almost all plant and animal foods—meat, eggs, nuts, grains, legumes, and vegetables. In fact, omega-6 fatty acids are so abundant in the diet that a deficiency isn't likely to ever happen. Less common are the omega-3 polyunsaturated fatty acids, but these can be found in seeds, leafy green vegetables, seaweed, eggs, fish, and shellfish. You can get all the omega-3 fatty acids you need by making sure you include some fish, eggs, and leafy greens as part of your weekly menu. Grass-fed beef and game meats also supply omega-3 fatty acids. Cattle that graze on grass, which is rich in omega-3s, incorporate these fats into their own tissues. Grain-fed beef, on the other hand, is a poor source of omega-3 fatty acids.

Macular Degeneration and Vegetable Oils

Macular degeneration is the most common irreversible cause of blindness in the U.S., affecting more than 10 million Americans. This isn't just an American problem; it's happening all over the world at an ever-increasing rate. As we age, our chances of developing macular degeneration increase dramatically. If you are over the age of 55, your chance of developing AMD is about one in ten, and those aren't good odds. Fortunately, medical research is showing that age-related macular degeneration may be preventable.

The major reason for blindness in the United States 40 years ago was diabetes, and age-related macular degeneration was rare. Today, AMD has overtaken diabetes fivefold and is now the leading cause of loss of vision in the United States as well as most other industrialized countries. Two-thirds of those who lose their vision are blind due to this condition.

"I've seen an exponential rise from the early 1970s through to the 1990s," says Dr. Paul Beaumont, an ophthalmologist and founding director of the Macular Degeneration Foundation of Australia. "If we look at Japan 40 years ago, the disease was rare; now it's common."

"I don't think there's any doubt we have an epidemic," says Dr. Beaumont, horrified by the rate at which AMD has multiplied and the fact that we've seen a tenfold increase in the last 30 years.

Although the disease progresses slowly, macular degeneration can affect eyesight very quickly. "One day I was doing crosswords and the next day I couldn't." says Jillian Price. For Jillian, the disease has disabled her life as an active woman. "Two months is very fast to lose so much sight; I've lost a lot of my independence," Ms. Price says. "Everything is distorted, getting on the buses [and] shopping is very hard, I can't read labels anymore."

For years researchers have sought for the cause and a cure. Recent research suggests that consuming coconut oil in place of other vegetable oils may help prevent this condition. Studies now show that if your diet includes soybean, corn, safflower, and other polyunsaturated vegetable oils, you may be at high risk for developing AMD. Polyunsaturated vegetable oil consumption has increased dramatically over the past 40 years as a result of fears about saturated fat. People have replaced the saturated fat in their diets with polyunsaturated fats believing it would reduce their risk of heart disease. Sadly, the expected results have not occurred, for heart disease is still the number one cause of death worldwide. However, this dramatic increase in the use of polyunsaturated vegetable oils has lead to an epidemic of age-related macular degeneration and is a likely suspect in cases of other degenerative eye diseases, especially those of the lens and the retina, which are most vulnerable to oxidative stress.

Over the past few years, several studies have linked polyunsaturated vegetable oils with macular degeneration.[21-22] The research shows that those people who use polyunsaturated vegetable oils in meal preparation are afflicted with the disease twice as commonly as those who don't. Even more convincing was a study in which those who ate a great deal of vegetable oil progressed toward macular degeneration at 3.8 times the rate of those who consumed only a little vegetable oil.[23] The risk of developing macular degeneration was lowest among those people who ate the most saturated fat, higher in those who at the greatest amount of monounsatured fat, and highest among those who ate the most polyunsaturated fat. Clearly, the greater the unsaturation of the oil, the higher the risk.

This makes sense, from a logical scientific perspective, because the more unsaturated an oil is, the more vulnerable it is to peroxidation and free-radical generation. Saturated fats are very resistant to peroxidation, so diets high in it increase the amount of this stable fat incorporated into eye tissue, which protects against lipid peroxidation associated with macular degeneration.

If you are concerned about eye and overall health, the oils you need to watch out for are the kind people tend to use every day: soybean, safflower, corn, and even canola oil, which is high in both monounsaturated and polyunsaturated fat. Be aware that this is not limited to your bottle of cooking oil or the oil you pour over your salad, as packaged convenience foods and junk foods are loaded with hidden polyunsaturated oils. Look at the ingredients in any sauce, dip, bread, cracker, cake mix, or frozen dinner, and you will find vegetable oils hidden in all of them. Unfortunately, most of us have been consuming these processed foods from the time we could walk.

"I think we could halve the number of people going blind with macular degeneration if we could change their diet and cut out the vegetable oil," Dr. Beaumont says.

Gwen Oliver, diagnosed with macular degeneration a few years ago, was astonished when Dr. Beaumont told her to steer clear of vegetable oils. "I was surprised about diet and all the products that we've been eating in the past," Oliver says. "We've always had it advertised that vegetable oil was far better for us."

Dr. Beaumont says he doesn't envision vegetable oils being removed from all foods, but says there should be a consumer health warning. "I think we have to have a warning on the packages similar to a warning of a cigarette package: 'Vegetable oil can lead to macular degeneration.'"

With the latest research pointing to vegetable oils as the main culprit, it may be possible to fend off this disease by simply changing our diets. The first step you should take to defend yourself from age-related macular degeneration is to eliminate most polyunsaturated oils, as well as foods made with them. Start by reading labels, particularly the ingredients list. The second step is to use coconut oil and other healthy saturated fats for most of your food preparation. The third step is to make sure you get plenty of fresh fruits and vegetables, which are high in antioxidant nutrients. The general recommendation is at least five servings per day.

Dr. Beaumont has lobbied the federal government to help fund awareness of this huge problem. "I think they should move fairly urgently," he says. "I don't think we can afford to delay in informing the public about something which can be affecting their vision." To date, however, nothing has happened. Fortunately, you do not need to wait for governmental intervention, which could take a long time, since economic and political factors are always at play. You can do something right now and take control of your health by carefully selecting the foods you put into your body.

Hydrogenated Vegetable Oils

Many packaged foods are made with hydrogenated or partially hydrogenated vegetable oil. These are among the most health-damaging fats you can possibly eat—just as bad, if not worse, than oxidized polyunsaturated fats.

Hydrogenated oils are made by bombarding liquid vegetable oil with hydrogen atoms in the presence of a metal catalyst. In the process, polyunsaturated vegetable oils become saturated with hydrogen. This forces the liquid oil to transform into a more viscous or solid fat. In the process of hydrogenation, however, a new type of fatty acid known as a trans fatty acid is created. Trans fatty acids are artificial man-made fats. This toxic fatty acid is foreign to our bodies and can create all sorts of trouble.

"These are probably the most toxic fats ever known," says Walter Willett, MD, Professor of Epidemiology and Nutrition at Harvard School of Public Health.[24] Studies show that trans fatty acids can contribute to atherosclerosis and heart disease. Trans fatty acids increase blood LDL (bad cholesterol) and lower the HDL (good cholesterol), both regarded to be undesirable changes.[25] Researchers now believe it has a greater influence on the risk of cardiovascular disease than any other dietary fat.[26]

Trans fatty acids affect more than just our cardiovascular health. They have been linked with a variety of adverse health effects, including cancer, MS, diverticulitis, diabetes, and other degenerative conditions.[27] Trans fatty acids disrupt brain communication. Studies show that the trans fatty acids we eat get incorporated into brain and eye cell membranes, including the myelin sheath that insulates neurons. Trans fatty acids alter the electrical activity of brain cells, causing cellular degeneration and diminished mental performance.[28]

Under pressure from many health organizations and the public, the United States Institute of Medicine spent three years reviewing all the published studies on trans fatty acids. After the study was completed, the Institute issued a statement declaring that no level of trans fatty acid consumption is safe. Surprisingly, the researchers provided no recommendation as to what percentage of trans fats are safe to consume, as is often done with food additives; rather they flatly stated that no trans fats are safe. If you see a packaged food that contains hydrogenated oil, margarine, or shortening, don't touch it. If you eat out, ask the restaurant manager what type of oil they use to cook their food. If they say, "Vegetable oil," it is almost definitely hydrogenated vegetable oil and should be avoided. Regular vegetable oil breaks down too quickly and becomes rancid, and restaurants like to reuse oil as long as possible before it is tossed out. Ordinary vegetable oils have too short a lifespan.

Many of the foods you buy in the store and in restaurants are prepared with or cooked in hydrogenated oil. Fried foods are usually cooked in hydrogenated oil because it makes foods crispy and is more resistant to spoilage than ordinary vegetable oils. Many frozen processed foods are cooked or prepared in hydrogenated oils, including French fries, biscuits, cookies, crackers, chips, pies, pizzas, peanut butter, cake frosting, and ice cream, especially soft serve. Most shortenings and margarines are produced using hydrogenated vegetable oils.

SATURATED FAT
Saturated Fat Is a Vital Nutrient

Probably no food component in history has been as misunderstood and maligned as saturated fat. It is accused of causing nearly every health problem of modern civilization. If it really is as dangerous as they say, it's truly a miracle that our ancestors managed to survive for so many thousands of years, since it was a mainstay in their diet. Animal fats, butter, and palm and coconut oils were the most common fats used throughout history. These fats are easy to produce using the simplest of tools. Vegetable oils from seeds such as soybean, cottonseed, safflower, and such are very difficult to extract. Consequently, polyunsaturated vegetable oils were not used much until after the invention of hydraulic oil presses in the 19th century. Interestingly enough, when people ate primarily saturated fats, the so-called diseases of modern civilization—heart disease, diabetes, Alzheimer's, glaucoma, and the like—were uncommon. As we've replaced saturated fats with unsaturated oils, these diseases have come upon us like a plague. From a historical point of view it is easy to see that saturated fats don't cause these diseases.

The truth of the matter is that saturated fat is a vital nutrient—yes, a nutrient and not at all the poison it is accused of being! It is necessary in order to obtain and maintain good health. Saturated fat serves as an important source of energy for the body and aids in the absorption of vitamins and minerals. As a food ingredient, fat helps us feel full and provides taste, consistency, and stability. Saturated fat is necessary for proper growth, repair, and maintenance of body tissues. It is essential for good lung function. It is the preferred source of energy for the heart muscle and also helps protect the unsaturated fats in your body against the destructive action of free radicals.

We hear a lot about the importance of the EFAs, and because "essential" is part of the name we have given them, we mistakenly believe they are the most important fats. However, the reason they are "essential" is because they are the least important of the fats. Believe it or not, saturated fat is far more important to your health than the EFAs! Let me explain why.

Saturated fat is so necessary to your health that our bodies have been programmed to make it out of other nutrients. Getting an adequate amount of saturated fat is so important and the consequences of a deficiency so severe that it is never left to chance. On the contrary, EFAs (polyunsaturated fats) are far less important so the body has not developed a means of manufacturing its own and can rely totally on dietary intake.

The foods we eat provide the building blocks for our cells and tissues. This is true for the fats we consume as well. The fat in our bodies consists of 45 percent saturated, 50 percent monounsaturated, and only 5 percent polyunsaturated. That's right, only 5 percent of the fat in your body is polyunsaturated. Consequently, the body's need for polyunsaturated fat or EFAs is very small. Your body needs nearly 10 times as much saturated fat, as well as monounsaturated fat, as EFA. Truly, which is more essential?

While the body can manufacture saturated and monounsaturated fats, it cannot make enough on its own for optimal health. We still need them in our diet to avoid nutritional deficiencies.[29-30]

Saturated Fat Does Not Promote Heart Disease

Reducing dietary saturated fat has generally been thought to improve cardiovascular health and protect against heart attacks and strokes. This assumption is based on the belief that dietary saturated fat increases blood cholesterol, thus promoting cardiovascular disease. However, blood cholesterol has little to do with heart disease; half of those people who suffer heart attacks have what is considered to be healthy and even optimal cholesterol levels. Obviously, having low cholesterol didn't help them any. Studies show that lowering cholesterol using drug therapy does not reduce heart attack deaths. Likewise, having high cholesterol does not increase the risk of experiencing a heart attack; in fact, studies show that women of all ages and men 60 years of age and over who have high cholesterol, actually live longer than those with lower cholesterol. A recent meta-analysis study published in *The American Journal of Clinical Nutrition* has conclusively proven that saturated fats are not harmful and do not cause or promote heart disease.[31]

Over the years, many studies have sought to prove the lipid hypothesis of heart disease—that diets high in saturated fat and cholesterol promote heart disease. Results have been mixed. Some seem to support this theory, while others do not. However, the majority of the medical community, along with the pharmaceutical industry (which profits greatly from the saturated fat-heart disease idea) supports the theory. Those studies that support the theory receive national press and are used as justification to establish government policies on health, while those that do not support the theory are generally ignored.

The simple fact is that the evidence in favor of the lipid hypothesis is no greater than the evidence that contradicts it. The number of studies for or against is not a major issue; some have involved relatively few participants, while others have used much larger numbers. Obviously, the results of a study involving 50,000 test subjects carries more weight than one involving only 1,000. One large study using 50,000 participants produces more reliable results than 10 small studies, with a total combined number of 10,000 participants. Therefore, the total number of studies is not as important as the number of people in the studies. If all the subjects in these many different studies were to be combined and evaluated equally, what would the final outcome be? Would it prove the lipid hypothesis or disprove it?

Researchers at the Children's Hospital Oakland Research Institute in California and Harvard School of Public Health got together to find out. They analyzed the highest-quality, most reliable studies over the past couple of decades that contained data for dietary saturated fat intake and risk of cardiovascular disease. Twenty-one studies were identified that fit their criteria. This meta-analysis study included data on nearly 350,000 subjects. With such a large subject database, the results would be far more reliable than any single study consisting of only 10,000 or even 100,000 subjects. The focus of the researchers was to determine if there is sufficient evidence linking saturated fat consumption to cardiovascular disease. Ultimately, those results indicated a resounding "no." The evidence proved that saturated fat intake is not associated with an increased risk of cardiovascular disease. Those subjects who ate the greatest amount of saturated fat were no more likely to suffer a heart attack or stroke than those who ate the least. It didn't matter how much saturated fat one ate, the incidence of heart disease was not affected.[31] This study gave definite proof using the highest-quality data available that saturated fats do not promote heart disease, thus clearly disproving the lipid hypothesis.

Since the publication of this landmark study in 2010, several others have been published confirming these results.[32-33] In 2014, researchers at the University of Cambridge published another, more extensive meta-analysis. This study included data from 72 previous studies with more than 600,000 participants from 18 nations. The results of the Cambridge study confirmed those of the Oakland Research Institute and Harvard study: People who eat the most saturated fat have no more incidence of heart disease than those who eat the least. In fact, the study discovered that some forms of saturated fat actually protect against heart disease.[34] The evidence is now clear: Saturated fats do not increase risk of heart disease and, in some cases, may even help prevent it.

These recent studies are not likely to change policies and recommendations about eating saturated fat anytime soon. Doctors have been warning us about the dangers of eating saturated fat for so many years that it is thoroughly ingrained into their minds, and they will likely continue to give this advice for many years, despite facts to the contrary. In other words, many health professionals will continue to ignore these studies and try to convince you to accept their opinions based on nothing more than a longstanding prejudice against saturated fat. The bottom line here is that you do not need to fear eating saturated fat or cholesterol, even if you hear criticism of them in the media or from your own doctor.

Top Nutrients for Good Eye Health

VITAMINS, MINERALS, AND PHYTONUTRIENTS

The nutrients in our foods can be divided into two major categories: energy-yielding and non-energy-yielding. Energy-yielding nutrients include fat (fatty acids), protein (amino acids), and carbohydrate (sugars). Each of these can be metabolized to produce energy, and that energy is measured in calories. Carbohydrate is the body's primary source of energy. Fat and protein can be used for energy, but they are also essential for building cells, tissues, and organs. The non-energy-yielding nutrients include vitamins, minerals, and phytonutrients (nutrients from plants); these provide no calories but are, nevertheless, vitally important to human health.

Vitamins are defined as organic compounds that are absolutely essential for normal growth, development, and function and are required in the diet because they cannot be synthesized by the body. Vitamin D is the only vitamin that doesn't conform completely with this general definition because it can be synthesized in the skin from exposure to sunlight.

Some vitamins are fat-soluble, such as vitamins A, D, E, and K, and are found in the fatty portion of plants and animals. Others are water-soluble, namely vitamin C and the B complex vitamins. The B complex vitamins are all related compounds that include thiamin (B1), riboflavin (B_2), niacin (B_3), vitamin B_6 (pyridoxine, pyridoxal, pyridoxamine), vitamin B_{12} (cobalamin), folate, pantothenic acid, and biotin.

Fat-soluble vitamins can be stored in the body for later use. We need these on a continual basis, but if we consume more than what is immediately needed, the excess is stored in the liver. This is beneficial in case there is a period of time when the vitamin may be lacking in the diet. However, if we consume too much, these vitamins can become toxic. This generally happens if a person takes too many supplements or eats a specially designed diet or formula diet that is exceptionally high in these vitamins. Under normal circumstances, you could not eat enough foods to create a toxicity.

Water-soluble vitamins do not collect in the body. Any excess is simply excreted, so you need to get an adequate amount of these vitamins every day.

There are many minerals that are vital to human health, some referred to as major minerals, are needed daily in milligram (mg) amounts and others, referred to a trace minerals, are needed only in very small amounts, micrograms (mcg). To give you an idea of the difference between these two measurements: 1 mg = 1000 mcg. An adult needs about 800 mg a day of calcium, one of the major minerals, but only about 70 mcg of selenium, a trace mineral. There are at least 16 major and trace minerals that are essential to human health and there may be others we need in very minute amounts for optimal health.

Vitamins and minerals are necessary for the proper, growth, development, repair, and maintenance of the human body. They function as part of the many thousands of enzymes and coenzymes that control nearly every chemical process in our bodies. Enzymes, for example, are not only necessary for digesting food, but are needed to convert glucose and fatty acids into energy within our cells. They control the synthesis of proteins and hormones, and are essential to proper function of the immune system, among many other things. Some enzymes function as powerful antioxidants to protect our cells and tissues from the destruction of free radicals. For example, antioxidant enzymes are necessary to protect the retina, lens, cornea, and all other eye tissues from harm.

In addition to vitamins and minerals, there are many other nutrients derived principally from plants (phytonutrients) that are also important for health. Some of the most notable are beta-carotene, alpha-carotene, lycopene, lutein, zeaxanthin, CoQ10, and rutin. Many of these belong to a class of phytonutrients known as carotenoids, which are fat-soluble; others are bioflavonoids, which are water-soluble. Although they are not considered essential and are, therefore, not classified as vitamins, many have shown to possess anti-inflammatory, antioxidant, antibacterial, antifungal, and anticancer properties, others improve blood circulation, speed tissue repair, help balance blood sugar, improve insulin secretion, and provide numerous other health benefits.

Essential vitamins and minerals have been studied and specific amounts have been determined to satisfy daily needs. This amount is known as the Recommended Dietary Allowance (RDA). An RDA for phytonutrients has not been set, however, in some cases a safe and adequate amount has been determined. The RDA is established to meet the needs for most healthy individuals, but if someone is under stress, exposed to environmental pollutants and toxins, consuming foods that contain chemical additives, sick, or suffering from chronic health problems (including chronic eye problems), the need for most vitamins and minerals is increased. Some nutrients offer better protection at levels higher than the RDA. For example, the RDA for vitamin C is a mere 60 mg, but most people will benefit from getting closer to 1000 mg per day.

A lack of good overall nutrition can promote premature aging and eye degeneration. For this reason, good nutrition is necessary for good eye health, as well as overall health. Some experts believe diet and lifestyle are the major contributing factors to poor eye health and with a proper diet, most common eye disorders such as cataracts, glaucoma, macular degeneration, and diabetic retinopathy can be prevented and to some extent possibly reversed.

VITAMIN A

Over the past few years, 55-year-old Alice, was finding it increasingly difficult to see at night. During the day she seemed to have no problem with her vision, but at night, in the dark, she became almost blind. Driving at night became more and more difficult and dangerous. Unless the streets were illuminated with bright lights, just staying on the road was a problem. Even when walking at night she would often bump into parked cars and benches.

Her medical history didn't indicate any obvious visual problems. She was not diabetic and was free of glaucoma, cataracts, and macular degeneration—the usual suspects. However, she had problems with Crohn's disease, an inflammatory bowel condition characterized by abdominal pain, diarrhea, and bleeding ulcers. She'd undergone three surgeries to remove portions of her bowel. She received regular vitamin B_{12} injections but no other supplementation. Her diet included lots of vegetables, but she smoked 10 cigarettes daily and drank occasionally.

Given her history of bowel surgeries, her doctor suspected that she might be suffering from a vitamin A deficiency, as removing portions of the intestinal tract can seriously reduce nutrient absorption. A blood test revealed that she was low in vitamin A. Normal vitamin A blood levels range from 1.5 to 4.2 micromole/l, and Alice's reading was only 0.3.

Initial treatment with oral vitamin A supplementation was ineffective in resolving the problem, indicating that the deficiency was not due to a dietary deficiency but related to malabsorption. Over the next 18 months, Alice made monthly visits to the clinic to receive vitamin A injections, and her night vision significantly improved.

Crohn's disease, ulcerative colitis, celiac disease, cystic fibrosis, pancreatic insufficiency, and intestinal surgery can all interfere with nutrient absorption. Bariatric surgery, also known as weight loss surgery, involves surgically removing a portion of the stomach to make it smaller, thus limiting the amount of food the patient can eat in order to facilitate weight loss. It can also lead to vitamin deficiencies. While vitamin A deficiency is relatively uncommon in affluent countries, the increasing rate of obesity may indirectly be leading to more cases.

Vitamin A deficiency can also be caused by malnutrition (not enough food) or a poor diet (eating the wrong types of food). Malnutrition is a common problem in many parts of the world where people often do not have enough to eat. A poor diet, which consists of eating the wrong types of food, can happen anywhere, including in more affluent countries because people often make unwise dietary choices that can lead to poor health.

Vitamin A is essential for good eye health, as it is necessary for the proper function of the cornea, conjunctiva, and retina. Among the complications associated with vitamin A deficiency are corneal and conjunctival xerosis (excessive dryness of the cornea and conjunctiva, producing irritation and itching) and keratomalacia (a softening and ulceration of the cornea). Vitamin A is a vital component of the retina and a deficiency can lead to a form of retinopathy called nyctalopia, or night blindness. Left untreated, these complications can lead to permanent visual loss. The gradual loss of night or dim-light vision is one of the first signs of a serious vitamin A deficiency.

Vitamin A deficiency manifesting as night blindness was recognized by the ancient Egyptians and Greeks. Doctors of the day advocated eating goat liver to restore vision and cure the condition. At the time, they did not know why liver would offer such curative powers, we now know that it is a rich source of vitamin A. Although there was no single event that can be called the "discovery" of vitamin A, it was the first of the fat-soluble vitamins to be identified and named. In the 19th century outbreaks of night blindness and corneal ulceration were linked to nutritional causes. In 1817 French physiologist, Francois Magendie conducted a series of experiments where he fed dogs a protein (and consequently a fat) deficient diet. The dogs lost weight, developed corneal ulcers, and subsequently died. Charles-Michel Billard reported similar corneal ulcers in abandoned, poorly fed infants under his care in Paris and remarked that the eye lesions resembled those in Magendie's protein- and fat-starved dogs. Corneal ulcers, often in association with night blindness, are now recognized as classic symptoms of vitamin A deficiency.

In the late 19th century the prevailing belief was that there were only four essential elements of nutrition: proteins, carbohydrates, fats, and minerals. Different proteins were considered of equal value in nutrition. Likewise, fats—whether from lard, butter, or cod liver oil—were considered equal in their nutritional properties. However, some investigators suggested that an unknown substance necessary for growth, one that supported life, was contained in milk and egg yolks, both sources of vitamin A.

In 1913 researchers showed that butter and egg yolks are not equivalent to other sources of fat, namely olive oil and lard in supporting the growth and survival of lab animals. When rats were fed a nutritionally deficient diet, butter and egg yolks kept them alive and healthy. However, when those were replaced with other fats, the animals' growth was stunted and their health declined. During World War I, malnourished children suffering from night blindness and corneal ulcers were cured when they were fed whole milk, butter, or cod liver oil. This life-saving, eyesight-restoring substance found in these foods became known as "fat-soluble A," a name that was shortened in 1920 to the one we know now as "vitamin A." Over the next couple of decades other essential vitamins were identified and were named vitamins B, C, D, and so forth.

Continued research has identified three forms of vitamin A: retinol, retinal, and retinoic acid. Transport proteins in the blood pick up vitamin A from the liver, where it is stored, and distributes it throughout the body. Special receptors on our cells pick up the vitamin. Each form of vitamin A triggers specific actions in the cells. Vitamin A is involved in several body processes. As stated, it is essential for producing good night vision as well as for the health of mucous membranes and skin, for growth of body tissues and bones, for maintaining stability of cell membranes, and for assisting in immune function. Notice that the various forms of vitamin A are all named in reference to the retina, attesting to the importance of this vitamin for good eyesight. Vitamin A is necessary to make the photopigment in the rod cells of the retina. This photopigment absorbs incoming light, triggering an electrical impulse that is sent down the retinal ganglion cell and to the brain. Rod cells allow us to see at night or in dim light, which is why a deficiency of this vitamin leads to the absence of photopigment and consequently, to night blindness.

Night blindness isn't the only effect vitamin A deficiency has on eyesight. When vitamin A is not present, the specialized cells that secrete mucus diminish in number and activity, and the cells of the mucous membranes, including those in the eye, change shape and begin to secrete keratin—the hard, inflexible protein of hair and nails. In the eye, the cornea becomes dry and hard and may develop ulcers, which may progress to permanent blindness.

Vitamin A is also found in the lens of the eye. One of its functions is that of an antioxidant, and it undoubtedly provides protection to the lens against free radicals.

Vitamin A deficiency is the number-one cause of childhood blindness in the world. It destroys the vision of half a million children each year, and another 5 million children worldwide suffer from less severe forms of vitamin A deficiency resulting in growth retardation and increased infections.

PROVITAMIN A CAROTENOIDS

We get vitamin A from fats in animal products. Good sources include beef liver, cod liver oil, oysters, whole milk, cream, cheese, butter, eggs, and fatty meat. You may have heard claims that carrots are good for the eyes because they contain vitamin A. Technically, this is not true, as only animal products contain vitamin A; however, plants do contain carotenoids, many of which can be converted by our bodies into vitamin A. In fact, the vitamin A we get from animals was once the carotenoids found in the grass, leaves, and other plants they ate. When these plants were eaten by an animal, some of the carotenoids were converted into vitamin A. Vitamin A tends to collect in fatty tissues.

Carotenoids are plant pigments that give red, yellow, orange, and green fruits and vegetables much of their color. The red color in tomatoes comes from carotenoids, as well as the orange color in carrots and cantaloupe. A carotenoid that can be converted into vitamin A is called provitamin A or vitamin A precursor. The efficiency in which carotenoids are transformed into vitamin A is low, so a much higher amount of carotenoids must be consumed to equal the amount of vitamin A you get from animal sources. Beta-carotene is the carotenoid that has the highest conversion rate. It takes about 12 times as much beta-carotene, by weight, to equal the amount of vitamin A from animal sources and about 24 times as much of the other carotenoids to do the same. There are about 50 known carotenoids in the human diet, but only a few can be converted into vitamin A. Other provitamin A carotenoids include alpha-carotene, gamma-carotene, and beta-cryptoxanthin. Most carotenoids, whether provitamin A carotenoids or not, function as antioxidants. Even if they aren't converted into vitamin A, they still provided important health benefits.

Foods that are good sources of carotenoids are fruits and vegetables with rich red, orange, yellow, and green colors such as leafy green vegetables (spinach, chard, turnip greens, bok choy, etc.), carrots, sweet potatoes, butternut squash, mangos, tomatoes, parsley, apricots, broccoli, red cabbage, and asparagus.

Unfortunately, eating foods rich in carotenoids is not necessarily enough to ward off vitamin A deficiency. Vitamin A is a fat-soluble nutrient. In order to effectively convert beta-carotene or any other provitamin A carotenoid into vitamin A, an adequate amount of fat must also be consumed at the same time. Eating beta-carotene with fat can improve the conversion rate sixfold.[1-2] In other words, you only need twice, rather than 12 times, as much beta-carotene to equal the amount of vitamin A you get in animal foods. Most vegetables and fruits do not contain enough fat for efficient conversion, so a person can eat large amounts of carotenoid-rich vegetables and fruits, yet still suffer from a vitamin A deficiency. For example, in Asia, many children eat diets containing what should be adequate amounts of provitamin A carotenoids, but due to poverty, they don't combine it with enough milk, eggs, and animal fat. Consequently, they suffer from vitamin A deficiency. They don't necessarily need to eat animal-based foods, which are often too costly, but adding vegetable-based fatty foods such as avocados, nuts, coconut, and oils such as palm, olive, and coconut would facilitate the conversion.

VITAMIN A REQUIREMENT

Many government health agencies have established a recommended dietary allowance for the essential nutrients. The U.S. government has set the RDA of vitamin A in adults at 900 mcg RAE (retinol activity equivalent) for men and 700 mcg RAE for women, 770 mcg RAE if pregnant and 1,300 mcg RAE if breastfeeding.

Our bodies convert all sources of vitamin A into the retinol form, so RAE is used in place of grams or other unites of measurement to account for the difference in the conversion rate of plant and animal sources; 1 RAE corresponds to the biological activity of 1 mcg of retinol, 2 mcg of beta-carotene with fat, 12 mcg of beta-carotene without fat, or 24 mcg of other provitamin A carotenoids.

To make it a little more confusing, you might see vitamin A measured in international units (IU). This system was used before the biological activity of vitamin A and carotenoids were fully understood. You will still see this form of measurement on supplements. For example, 900 mcg RAE equals 6,000 IU of beta-carotene in supplement form.

Since vitamin A is an essential nutrient and is required for normal eye function, some people might assume that if a little is good, more might be better and consume large quantities in an attempt to prevent or treat some eye or health condition. You can't overdose on vitamin

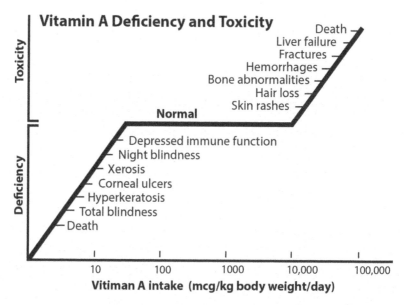

Deficiency symptoms occur from zero up to approximately 50 mcg/ kg. Sufficient vitamin A levels continue from there to about 10,000 mcg/kg. More than this leads to toxicity symptoms. For reference, 100 mcg/kg of body weight would equal about 7,000 RE for a 150 pound (70kg) person. Adapted from Hathcock, J. Vitamin safety: A current appraisal. Vitamin Issues 1985;5:4.

A by eating plant sources because carotenoids will only be converted as needed by the body.[3] However, you can get too much if you eat a lot of liver or take an excessive amount of dietary supplements.

Your body will function best if you provide a little vitamin A every day, however, too much at one time or over a period of time can become toxic. Because vitamin A is fat soluble, the body stores any excess in the liver. This is why liver is such a good dietary source. Too much vitamin A can lead to skin irritation, hair loss, joint and bone pain, fractures, liver failure, and death. Not enough vitamin A, on the other hand, can lead to night blindness, xerosis (excessively dry mucous membranes), corneal ulcers, hyperkeratosis (thickening and hardening of the skin), total blindness, and death. There is a happy medium in which the body receives enough of the vitamin to prevent deficiency disease but not so much as to become toxic. Fortunately, there is a wide range that separates deficiency from toxicity.

ANTIOXIDANTS

Studies have repeatedly shown that much of the damage occurring in the eyes from the various eye disorders is caused by oxidation of fats and proteins and the formation of destructive free radicals. Our bodies keep a reserve of antioxidant enzymes and nutrients on hand to fight off and neutralize free radicals. However, if free radicals form faster than the available antioxidants can quench them, a state of oxidative stress occurs. When this happens, tissues and cells are damaged.

Oxidative stress can occur if we are exposed to an extraordinarily high influx of free radicals or we don't consume enough antioxidant nutrients on a regular basis. The major antioxidants important to eye health are: vitamins A, C, and E; the carotenoids beta-carotene, lycopene, lutein, zeaxanthin, and astaxanthin; and the minerals zinc and selenium. If a lack of adequate antioxidants is to blame for the tissue breakdown associated with the various eye disorders, then a seemingly simple answer might be to consume more foods or supplements that provide these antioxidants.

This idea has been heavily researched over the past several decades, and the results have been both encouraging and disappointing. Some studies show that adding antioxidant supplements into the diet slow down the progression and reduce the risk of developing cataracts, glaucoma, macular degeneration, and retinopathy. Dietary studies in which participants ate foods rich in antioxidants gave similar results. However, other studies have shown no benefit. This discrepancy has baffled researchers.

One possible reason for the discrepancy is the source of the antioxidants. Dietary supplements generally consist of synthetically produced nutrients that may not provide the same degree of protection as natural nutrients. In addition, supplements generally consist of only one or just a few isolated nutrients. Foods provide a wide range of nutrients that generally work synergistically with each other to improve their efficiency. For example, a supplement of beta-carotene would contain only beta-carotene, while beta-carotene-rich foods also contain alpha-, gamma-, and delta-carotene and a variety of other carotenoids and nutrients that could enhance their antioxidant and health promoting properties. There are about 50 different carotenoids in our foods, and supplements provide only one or two. There are eight varieties of Vitamin E but only one, alpha tocopherol, is generally ever used in supplements, even though some of the other forms are much more effective antioxidants. Some nutrients improve the absorption of others. For example, vitamin C increases the absorption of chromium and iron. Some nutrients, taken in large, isolated doses (as in the case of supplements), can interfere with the absorption of other nutrients. For instance, large doses of vitamin A can interfere with the absorption of vitamin K. Likewise, large doses of alpha-tocopherol, the most common form of vitamin E, can compete with and interfere with the absorption of other forms of vitamin E.[4] Eating real foods provide a more balanced source of nutrients.

Another major reason for the conflicting results is the nutritional status of the study participants. If a person is experiencing symptoms of night blindness as a result of a vitamin A deficiency, for example, supplying the missing vitamin can correct the problem. However, if the problem is actually a zinc deficiency, which is needed to transport vitamin A to the retina, no amount of vitamin A will correct the problem; in this case, zinc is what is needed. Poor night vision can also occur as a result of a genetic condition called retinitis pigmentosa or as a consequence of cataracts or diabetic retinopathy. If a vitamin A deficiency isn't present, then giving the affected person more vitamin A simply will not help.

One of the shortcomings of these antioxidant studies is the assumption or hope that the nutrients can provide a pharmaceutical or therapeutic effect above just satisfying a nutrient deficiency. However, studies suggest that antioxidant supplementation is most beneficial when the subjects are poorly nourished or are experiencing nutrient deficiencies. When subjects are well nourished, supplementation is generally ineffective.[5]

For instance, in two similar cancer prevention studies using nutritional supplements, end-of-study eye examinations were conducted to assess the effect of the supplements on cataract prevalence. One study noted no effect of either vitamin E or beta-carotene on cataract prevalence after supplementing the diet for a average of 6.6 years.[6] However, the other study, conducted in a nutritionally deprived population, noted a beneficial effect for cataracts with the use of multivitamin and mineral supplements (containing vitamin E and beta-carotene) after 5 to 6 years.[7]

If a person is deficient in vitamin E, supplying him or her with an adequate amount of the nutrient may bring improvement or at least slow down the progress of the disease. If there is no vitamin E deficiency, giving more of the vitamin will not be helpful, and too much can become harmful. This is true with vitamin A, vitamin E, and with most other antioxidant nutrients.

Studies indicate that antioxidant nutrients can significantly reduce the risk of age-related macular degeneration, cataracts, and other degenerative eye diseases. People with low blood levels of key antioxidants like vitamins E and C are at risk. Increasing blood levels of these nutrients reduces the risk, but increasing the levels beyond a point offers no additional beneficial effect.[8]

Everyone has a different need when it comes to antioxidant nutrients. Those who are exposed to a lot of environmental pollutants, are under heavy stress, or eat a lot of sugar or polyunsaturated vegetable oils need higher levels of antioxidants.

LUTEIN AND ZEAXANTHIN

Most people would probably benefit from increasing the antioxidant content of their diets because we generally don't get enough of these nutrients on a daily basis. Two such antioxidant nutrients many are deficient in are lutein and zeaxanthin. Of all the carotenoids found in the human diet, only a small few are able to pass through the blood brain barrier, the most notable are lutein and zeaxanthin. These are the only carotenoids normally found in the retina and serve an essential function. Their importance in protecting and maintaining good eye health has gained them a reputation as superstars for ocular nutrition.

These nutrients have shown to be especially useful in protecting against retinal diseases such as macular degeneration. For instance, researchers at Harvard Medical School evaluated dietary intake of a variety of antioxidant nutrients, including several carotenoids, vitamins A, C, and E, and their relationship to the risk of AMD. Lutein and zeaxanthin were, by far, the most protective, just 6 mg per day reduced risk by an impressive 43 percent.[9]

Studies have also shown that lutein and zeaxanthin can prevent retinal damage and preserve visual function in cases of diabetic retinopathy, even when blood sugar levels are not well controlled.[10]

Both lutein and zeaxanthin are necessary for good eye function. They serve an essential function in the retina. At the center of the macula is a depression called the fovea (see diagram on page 15). The fovea contains the largest concentration of photoreceptor cone cells, which are responsible for both detailed and color vision. Light from our forward vision focuses on the fovea and macula. Consequently, this area of the retina receives the greatest intensity of incoming light and the greatest exposure to high-energy wavelengths of light that generate free radicals. Without some protection, the retina would quickly degenerate and lose its ability to function properly. Fortunately, the macula contains a protective substance known as macular pigment, that prevents much of the harmful effects of sunlight. Macular pigment is comprised of three known compounds: lutein, zeaxanthin, and meso-zeaxanthin.

Lutein and zeaxanthin are orange-yellow pigments that give plants such as yellow squash, orange bell peppers, corn, and marigold flowers their distinctive colors, but they are also found in red, orange, and dark green fruits and vegetables. Meso-zeaxanthin is not found in the diet but is produced in the retina from lutein. It is the most potent antioxidant of the three, but is only found in the center portion of the macula, where vision is sharpest. There are five times more of these carotenoids in the macula than in the rest of the surrounding retina. There is more zeaxanthin in the fovea than lutein, but in the periphery, zeaxanthin declines more rapidly than lutein, so lutein becomes dominant.

The high density of lutein and zeaxanthin in the fovea and the 3-4 mm area surrounding it colors this part of the retina yellow. The name of this area, *macula lutea*, in Latin means "yellow spot." It is generally referred to simply as the "macula."

Macular pigment absorbs much of the damaging high-energy blue light that enters the eye. Blue wavelengths of visible light produce the most oxidative stress in the retina. Exposure to blue light over a lifetime can contribute substantially to the development of age-related macular degeneration. Studies show that low dietary intake of lutein and zeaxanthin results in lower levels in the macula, which can degrade vision and increase risk of macular degeneration.

The benefits of lutein and zeaxanthin are not limited to the retina, for the health of the lens also depends on them. In addition to vitamins A and E, lutein and zeaxanthin are present in the lens. There is a reason for this. The lens is also subjected to high-energy wavelengths of light and, therefore, needs constant antioxidant protection. These antioxidants provide that protection. Studies have shown a lower incidence of cataracts with higher intake levels of lutein and zeaxanthin.[11]

While studies of antioxidant nutrients have produced mixed results as to their effectiveness against degenerative eye diseases in general, most studies with lutein and zeaxanthin have produced positive results. One of the reasons may be that we don't eat enough of the foods that contain these nutrients. Some of the best sources are dark green leafy vegetables such as spinach, kale, and collard greens. People who avoid vegetables are likely deficient in these important carotenoids. Egg yolks are another good source, but the misguided fear of cholesterol over the past few decades has compelled people to shy away from eating whole eggs and consume only the whites. This is a big mistake, based on a faulty premise. Egg whites contain neither of these important carotenoids, but yolk is one of the richest dietary sources of both lutein and zeaxanthin; in fact, these carotenoids give the yolk its distinctive yellow color. The darker and richer the color, the higher the carotenoid content. This is one reason why eggs from free-range chickens that have access to growing grass and other plants have richer-colored yolks.

In a study published in *The British Journal of Ophthalmology*, an international team of researchers analyzed the carotenoid content of 33 common caroteniod-rich foods. Egg yolks and corn (maize) came out on the top of the list as the richest combined source of lutein and zeaxanthin, comprising more than 85 percent of their total carotenoid content. The richest source of lutein was corn, followed by egg yolks, kiwi, pumpkin, zucchini, and spinach. The richest source of zeaxanthin was orange bell pepper, followed by egg yolks and corn.

Lutein is far more common in foods than zeaxanthin. Two-thirds (22) of the foods tested were good sources of lutein, while only eight of the 33 were equally as good for zeaxanthin. Most of the dark green leafy vegetables often recommended as good sources of lutein and zeaxanthin had 15 to 47 percent of their carotenoids as lutein but a very low content (0 to 3 percent) of zeaxanthin.[12] The table on the following page shows relative amounts of the major carotenoids in

Carotenoids in Select Foods

Food	Lutein and zeaxanthin	Lutein	Zeaxanthin	Cryptoxanthins	Alpha-carotene	Beta-carotene
Egg Yolk	89	54	35	4	0	0
Corn	86	60	25	5	0	0
Kiwi	54	54	0	0	0	8
Red Seedless Grapes	53	43	10	4	3	16
Zucchini Squash	52	47	5	24	0	5
Pumpkin	49	49	0	0	0	21
Spinach	47	47	0	19	0	16
Orange Pepper	45	8	37	22	8	21
Yellow Squash	44	44	0	0	28	9
Cucumber	42	38	4	38	0	4
Pea	41	41	0	21	0	5
Green Pepper	39	36	3	20	0	12
Red Grape	37	33	4	29	1	6
Butternut Squash	37	37	0	34	5	0
Orange Juice	35	15	20	25	3	8
Honeydew	35	17	18	0	0	48
Celery	34	32	2	40	13	0
Green Grapes	31	25	7	52	0	7
Brussels Sprouts	29	27	2	39	0	11
Scallions	29	27	3	35	0	0
Green Beans	25	22	3	42	1	5
Orange	22	7	15	12	8	11
Broccoli	22	22	0	49	0	27
Apple (Red Delicious)	20	19	1	23	5	17
Mango	18	2	16	4	0	20
Green Lettuce	15	15	0	36	16	0
Tomato Juice	13	11	2	2	12	16
Peach	13	5	8	8	10	50
Yellow Pepper	12	12	0	1	1	0
Nectarine	11	6	6	23	0	48
Red Pepper	7	7	0	2	24	3
Tomato	6	6	0	0	0	12
Carrots	2	2	0	0	43	55
Cantaloupe	1	1	0	0	0	87
Dried Apricots	1	1	0	9	0	87
Green Kidney Beans	0	0	0	28	0	0

Carotenoid content is given in mole%. Adapted from: Sommerburg, O, et al. Fruits and vegetables that are sources for lutein and zeaxanthin: the macular pigment in human eyes. *Br J Ophthalmol* 1998;82:907-910.

the 33 foods tested. Also included in the table are crytoxanthin, alpha-carotene, and beta-carotene, which are vitamin A precursors.

Another antioxidant carotenoid that is very similar to lutein and zeaxanthin is astaxanthin. It, too, can pass through the blood brain barrier and directly affect the eyes. Astaxanthin is the pigment responsible for the red color in salmon, lobster, krill, crab, and other shellfish. It is found in the micro algae *Haematoccous pluvialis*, which is eaten by marine animals and gives them their distinctive coloring.

Astaxanthin is a much more powerful antioxidant than beta-carotene, alpha-tocopherol (vitamin E), zeaxanthin, and lutein. Studies indicate that it is 14 times more potent than vitamin E, 54 times more potent than beta-carotene, and 65 times more potent than vitamin C in scavenging free radicals.

Dr. Mark Tso, of the Wilmer Eye Institute at Johns Hopkins University, has shown that astaxanthin easily crosses into the tissues of the eye and exerts its effects with more potency than lutein or zeaxanthin, with no adverse reactions. Astaxanthin has the potential to ameliorate or prevent light-induced damage, photoreceptor cell damage, ganglion cell damage, and damage to the neurons of the inner retinal layers. Tso claims that astaxanthin supplementation could be effective in preventing or treating a number of eye diseases that involve oxidative stress, including: AMD, diabetic neuropathy, cystoid macular edema, central retinal arterial and venous occlusion, glaucoma, and inflammatory eye diseases (i.e., retinitis, iritis, keratitis, scleritis, etc.).

Astaxanthin is emerging as a preeminent antioxidant dietary supplement for general health as well as for the prevention and mitigation of degenerative diseases of the eye. Unless you eat a lot of salmon or shellfish, you are probably not getting much astaxanthin in your diet.

The best source for all antioxidants is food, just like any other nutrient. However, sometimes it can be of benefit to boost the amount or supplement what you get in foods with an oral supplement.

There is no established RDA for lutein, zeaxanthin, or astaxanthin nor are there any known toxic side effects from taking unusually large amounts (up to 70 mg). So they are considered quite safe. The amounts of lutein and zeaxanthin used in most human clinical trials range from 6 to 20 mg per day. Multivitamin supplements normally do not contain these nutrients, and if they do, the amount is generally small, around 0.25 mg per tablet. Some experts recommend that we should get at least 6 mg of lutein per day in order to achieve beneficial effects. If you take a dietary supplement, check the label; if the amount is listed in mcgs, this refers to micrograms, not milligrams (mg). It takes 1,000 mcg to equal 1 mg. Also, if the ingredient is listed as a combination lutein/zeaxanthin, know that the amount of zeaxanthin is only about 1/20th of the amount indicated. Krill oil is a popular source for astaxanthin with 2 mg per day being generally recommended.

At this time, the lutein, zeaxanthin, and astaxanthin found in supplements are not synthesized in some chemist's lab, but come from plants and animals. Sources for lutein are generally marigold flower petals, while zeaxanthin is taken from paprika or red peppers. Astaxanthin comes from algae or krill.

VITAMIN C AND GLUCOSE

Vitamin C is one of our major antioxidants. It can also reactivate the antioxidant activity of vitamin E after it has used up its antioxidant ability neutralizing free radicals. In addition to being a potent antioxidant, vitamin C is necessary for the production of thyroid hormones, for amino acid metabolism, to strengthen the immune system, and to synthesize collagen—the fibrous, structural protein in connective tissues. Collagen serves as the matrix on which bone and teeth are formed and gives strength and elasticity to our skin and organs. Our cells are held together largely by collagen; this is especially important in the capillaries and the artery walls, which must expand and contract with each heartbeat. A lack of vitamin C can weaken blood vessels and capillaries allowing them to break and leak.

Many researchers recommend increasing antioxidant consumption to help reduce the risk of age-related eye disorders. Most of us would benefit from more of these protective antioxidants, but a lack of dietary antioxidants isn't the only factor that can lead to antioxidant deficiency. Antioxidant depletion increases with exposure to pollution and toxins, eating polyunsaturated oils, consuming too many calories, and eating excessive amounts of sugar and carbohydrate.

If you eat more than 200 mg of carbohydrate in a day (300 mg is typical), mostly from refined grains and sugar, and do not eat much fresh fruit or vegetables, it is almost guaranteed that you are deficient in Vitamin C. This is important to correct, because vitamin C reactivates vitamin E, and therefore, a vitamin C deficiency can lead to a vitamin E deficiency, thereby greatly increasing the risk of oxidative stress so common in all major eye disorders.

When you eat large amounts of refined carbohydrate you can create a vitamin C deficiency, even if you are consuming the RDA of vitamin C (in the U.S. it is 60 mg/day). If you are diabetic or pre-diabetic, your need for vitamin C is even greater because your high blood levels of glucose reduces the amount of vitamin C your tissues absorb.

Glucose and vitamin C molecules are very similar in structure. Most animals can generate their own vitamin C from glucose derived from the carbohydrates in their diets. Humans, however, cannot. We do not have the enzymes to make this conversion, so we must get our vitamin C directly from the foods we eat. The similarity between glucose and vitamin C extends beyond the molecular structure; it also includes the way they are attracted to and enter cells. Both molecules require help from insulin before they can penetrate cell membranes.

Glucose and vitamin C compete with each other for entry into our cells, but it is not really a fair competition. Our bodies favor glucose entry at the expense of vitamin C. When blood glucose levels are elevated, vitamin C absorption into the cells is severely restricted. Whenever you eat a meal that contains carbohydrate, it will be converted into glucose, which will interfere with vitamin C absorption. The more carbohydrate you eat, the higher your blood glucose goes, and the less vitamin C your body utilizes. It is ironic that you can drink sweetened orange juice or sugary breakfast cereals that are fortified with extra vitamin C, yet the sugar in these products almost completely blocks the absorption of the vitamin. A high-carbohydrate diet can lead to vitamin C deficiency. If a person is diabetic or insulin resistant, even a little, blood glucose is elevated for extended periods of time, blocking vitamin C absorption even more.

For this reason, diets high in carbohydrate can cause vitamin C deficiency and, consequently, low thyroid function and other problems. The effect of carbohydrate on blocking the absorption of vitamin C is highly significant, yet generally unrecognized by most doctors. It is possible to develop severe vitamin deficiency even when the diet contains what we might consider ample sources of vitamin C.

Severe vitamin C deficiency leads to scurvy, which may include any of the following: anemia, depression, frequent infections, bleeding gums, loose teeth, muscle degeneration and pain, joint pain, slow healing of wounds and injuries, degeneration of collagen, and the development of atherosclerosis (hardening of the arteries), which can lead to heart attacks and strokes. Scurvy can eventually lead to death. It is far more likely for you to suffer a heart attack or stroke from eating a vitamin C-robbing, high-carbohydrate diet than by eating a high-fat diet.

OMEGA-3 FATTY ACIDS

Two omega-3 long chain polyunsaturated fatty acids needed for good brain and eye health are eicosapentaenoic acid (EPA) and docosahexaenoic acid (DHA). Both of these can be synthesized in our bodies from alpha-linolenic acid, the type of omega-3 fatty acid found in flaxseed and other plants. However, this complex, multistep process requires many enzymes to complete. While alpha-linolenic acid can be converted into EPA and DHA, less than 10 percent of this omega-3 fatty acid actually completes the conversion process. A better source of these two important omega-3 long chain fatty acids is fish. Fish contains both EPA and DHA, so no conversion is necessary. When you eat 1 gram of fish-derived EPA or DHA, you get essentially 1 gram. When you eat 1 gram of alpha-linolenic acid, you only get 0.1 gram of EPA/DHA, at best.

Of these two, DHA is of particular importance to the brain and eyes. The brain contains more DHA than any other part of our body. In the eye, the photosensitive rods and cones of the retina contain the highest percentage of this long chain omega-3 fatty acid. The outer segments of the rods and cones consist of stacks of membranous disks (see diagram on page 18). New disks are continually produced to replace old disks. Shedding of the disks occurs at the tips of the photoreceptors as they are exposed to light during the normal day and night cycle. Rods shed and renew their entire outer column of disks every 9 to 12 days. Cones also shed their disks, but in a less synchronized manner and at a slightly slower rate. In both cases, the layer of retinal pigment adjacent to the tips of the rods and cones captures the discarded segments and digests them.

EPA and DHA are highly unstable chemically, and therefore, extremely vulnerable to lipid peroxidation. When exposed to light, they spontaneously oxidize and generate hydrogen peroxide free radicals. This chemical reaction is involved in the process of generating visual signals that are sent from the retina to the optic nerve, but during the process, the outer disks of the photoreceptors are damaged and must be continually replaced. Once free radicals are formed, they attack surrounding molecules and transform them into free radicals as well. Antioxidants are needed to block these reactions. Since the retina is a hotbed of free-radical activity, it must have an abundance of antioxidants for protection. This is why eating a diet high in antioxidant nutrients is so important to good eye health. It is ironic that we need DHA for sight, but it also instigates much of the potentially damaging free-radical activity that occurs in the eye.

In order for the photoreceptors to function properly, there must be a constant source of long chain omega-3 fatty acids available. A deficiency of these fatty acids could seriously affect the function of the retina. Consequently, many studies have sought to investigate the relationship between the consumption of omega-3 fatty acids and eye disorders, in particular macular degeneration. The results have been mixed. Some studies seem to show that higher fish or fish oil consumption reduces risk of macular degeneration or diabetic retinopathy, while others indicate no effect.[13] Some studies have even shown a detrimental effect, with accelerated degeneration of the retina.[14]

When consumed, omega-3 fatty acids are incorporated into cellular membranes throughout the body and find their way into many structures in the eye, not only the cones and rods. Too many of these fatty acids can affect the function of the cell membranes and, because of their high vulnerability to oxidation, can be the source of a great deal of free-radical activity. As is the case with many other important nutrients, we need some for good health, but too many can become detrimental or toxic. It is likely that the conflicting results in the studies are due to the subjects' omega-3 status. If the subjects were deficient in omega-3, consumption of fish or supplementation with fish oil would be beneficial. For those who were not deficient, there would be no significant benefit or perhaps even a detrimental effect if given too much.

While there is a wide range of values between deficiency and toxicity with many essential vitamins and minerals, the window with omega-3 fatty acids is much narrower. The requirement for alpha-linolenic acid is 0.4 percent of calories consumed or about 1 gram a day.[15] This is the amount you would get from a single 1 gram capsule.

The problem with fish and flaxseed oil supplements is that they degrade very quickly. As soon as the fatty acids are extracted and bottled or encapsulated, they begin to degrade. To complicate the matter, you really have no idea how old the supplements are when you purchase them. If they are not refrigerated, the degeneration occurs faster. For this reason, it is best to get your omega-3 fatty acids from real food, which is always the best source of nutrients. You can get omega-3 fatty acids from leafy green vegetables, sea vegetables (kelp, nori, etc.), fish and shellfish, and eggs. Eating one to two servings of fish a week is generally recommended for adequate omega-3 intake.

A DAILY DOSE OF ANTIOXIDANTS
FROM A COOKING OIL

According to the WHO, 250 million children worldwide suffer from vitamin A deficiency, with thousands of children going blind and dying each year as a result. Millions more suffer from subclinical vitamin A deficiency; in other words, they consume enough vitamin A to prevent serious deficiency symptoms like corneal ulcers but not enough for proper growth and development or to prevent night blindness. Most of these children live in Asia and sub-Saharan Africa.

Health authorities in the affected countries have tried to find economically feasible solutions to this problem. They have tried dispersing dietary supplements and increasing the consumption of provitamin A-rich produce, but costs and other difficulties have limited their success. However, several governments have now found a potentially suitable answer—red palm oil.

Palm oil comes from the fruit of the oil palm, which is totally different from the type of palm that produces coconuts. Palm fruit is about the size of a small plum. The oil is extracted from the fibrous fruit surrounding the seed. Palm fruit is a dark red color and produces an orange-red colored oil. This crude or virgin oil is called red palm oil. Red palm oil has undergone minimal processing and retains most of the naturally occurring fat-soluble vitamins and other nutrients. The distinctive red color comes from the rich abundance of beta-carotene and other carotenoids in the fruit.

Red palm oil is a virtual powerhouse of nutrition. It contains far more nutrients than any other dietary oil. It is the richest dietary source of beta-carotene and alpha-carotene—both vitamin A precursors. It has 15 times more beta-carotene than carrots and 44 times more than that found in leafy vegetables. In addition, it contains lycopene, gamma-carotene, lutein, and some 20 other carotenes, along with vitamins E and K, CoQ10, phytosterols, flavonoids, phenolic acids, and glycolipids. Palm oil is packed with all the different forms of vitamin E, including a very special form of called tocotrienol. There are four different types of tocotrienols, and palm oil contains all of them. These tocotrienols have up to 60 times the antioxidant power as ordinary vitamin E (alpha-tocopherol). The combination of vitamin E (tocopherols), tocotrienols, carotenes, and other antioxidants makes red palm oil a natural, super-potent antioxidant food, so much so that it is currently being encapsulated and sold as a vitamin supplement. The oil is also available in bottles, like other vegetable oils, for kitchen use.

Governments around the world are now instigating programs to include red palm oil in cookies, breads, and other baked goods to provide children suffering from vitamin A deficiency with an inexpensive source of the important vitamin. Nursing mothers can eat it to enhance the vitamin A content in their milk. Red palm oil solves one of the problems children and nursing mothers face in some of the poorest areas of the world. While they may have access to carotenoid-rich vegetables, they often don't get enough fat in their diets to properly convert carotenoids into vitamin A. However, the provitamin A carotenoids in red palm oil come with their own source of oil, thus greatly enhancing carotenoid conversion and absorption. The oil palm is native to many parts of Africa and is cultivated throughout South-east Asia, so it provides an economically feasible and readily available dietary source of vitamin A that can solve the massive worldwide problem of vitamin A deficiency.

Red palm oil provides an excellent natural source of protective antioxidants. It contains a full spectrum of them, not only the few you'll get in the average multivitamin. Red palm is the best natural source of the super-potent form of vitamin E (tocotrienols). Tocotrienols have shown to help protect against heart disease and stroke by maintaining proper blood pressure. This powerful antioxidant also inhibits platelets from sticking to one another, thereby naturally thinning the blood. It also reduces inflammation and assists in keeping blood vessels properly dilated so circulation remains normal and blood pressure stays under control.

In one study, researchers induced inflammation in the arteries of test animals. Inflammation causes swelling, narrowing artery passageways and restricting blood flow to vital organs such as the heart. Half of the animals received tocotrienols in their diet, while the other half served as the control. In the control group artery passageways were severely constricted and 42 percent of the animals died. However, those who received the tocotrienols showed far less inflammation and constriction, resulting in a 100 percent survival rate.

Tocotrienols strengthen the heart so it can better withstand stress. Researchers can purposely induce heart attacks in lab animals by cutting off blood flow to the heart. This causes severe injury and death. However, if the animals are fed tocotrienol-rich palm oil beforehand, survival rate is greatly increased, injury is minimized, and recovery time is reduced.[16]

The antioxidant power of palm oil has also shown to be of benefit in protecting against neurological degeneration. Two of the most significant factors that affect brain function are oxidative stress and poor circulation. Researchers have found correlations between oxidative stress and reduced blood flow to the brain to senile dementia, Alzheimer's disease, Parkinson's disease, and even schizophrenia, all of which involve brain cell death. Tocotrienols aid the brain by reducing oxidative stress and improving blood flow.

Researchers can mimic much of the destruction seen in the above neurological disorders by feeding test animals large doses of glutamate, which kills brain cells. The primary action of cell death is caused by free radicals. Ordinary vitamin E is not strong enough to prevent glutamate-induced cell death, but palm tocotrienols can quench the destructive action of glutamate. In laboratory studies tocotrienol-treated neurons maintained healthy growth and motility, even in the presence of excess glutamate.[17]

Research shows that tocotrienols can be of help with a number of common health problems including osteoporosis, asthma, cataracts, macular degeneration, arthritis, and liver disease, as well as stunting the processes that promote premature aging.

One tablespoon supplies more than enough to meet daily requirements of vitamins E and A. The best way to take red palm oil is to incorporate it into daily food preparation, using it like any other cooking oil. It is very heat stable and is excellent for cooking and baking.

Because of its distinctive orange-red color, red palm oil is easy to spot on store shelves. At room temperature it is semisolid, somewhat like soft butter. If refrigerated, it will harden. On the countertop on a warm day, it will liquefy. Red palm oil doesn't need to be refrigerated; it is very resistant to oxidation. You can use the oil when it is hard or soft. Nutritionally, there is no difference.

Red palm oil has a distinctive flavor and aroma. In cultures where it is produced, it is an important ingredient in food preparation and gives the food much of its characteristic flavor. The oil has a pleasant, somewhat savory taste that enhances the natural flavor of meats and vegetables. It also complements soups, sauces, sautéed vegetables, eggs, and meats. In recipes that call for vegetable oil, shortening, or margarine, red palm oil makes for an excellent, healthy replacement.

Palm fruit produces two types of oil; one from the fleshy fruit and the other from the seed or kernel. Red palm oil comes from the soft fruit, while palm kernel oil is extracted from the seed. The two are not alike. Palm kernel oil is almost identical to coconut oil, colorless and contains about 53 percent MCTs. Red palm oil contains no MCTs, but it provides a rich source of antioxidants.

Red palm oil is available at most good health food stores and online. To learn more about the many health benefits of tocotrienols and palm oil, I recommend my book, *The Palm Oil Miracle*.

FAT INTAKE AND NUTRIENT ABSORPTION

Dietary fat is an important part of a healthy eating plan and can have a significant effect on eye health. Low-fat diets actually accelerate eye aging and increase the risk of developing age-related degenerative eye disease.

Adding fat to your food slows down the movement of the food through your stomach and digestive system. This is a good thing because it allows more time for foods to bathe in stomach acids and digestive enzymes. As a consequence, more nutrients, including protective antioxidant nutrients that may be tightly bound to other compounds, are released from the foods and made available for absorption into the body.

Low-fat diets prevent complete digestion of food and limit nutrient absorption, promoting nutrient deficiencies. Calcium, for example, needs fat for proper absorption. For this reason, low-fat diets encourage osteoporosis. It is interesting that we often avoid fat as much as possible and eat low-fat foods, including non-fat and low-fat milk for calcium; yet, calcium is not effectively absorbed from reduced-fat milk. This may be one of the reasons why people can drink loads of milk and take calcium supplements by the handful but still suffer from osteoporosis. Likewise, many vegetables are good sources of calcium, but in order to take advantage of that calcium, you need to eat them with butter and cream or other foods that contain fat.

Fat improves the availability and absorption of almost all vitamins and minerals and is essential for the proper absorption of fat-soluble nutrients: vitamins A, D, E, and K, as well as alpha-carotene, beta-carotene, lycopene, lutein, zeaxanthin, and other carotenoids. These nutrients are absolutely vital to good eye health.

Many fat-soluble vitamins function as antioxidants that protect your eyes from free-radical damage. By reducing the amount of fat in your diet, you limit the amount of protective antioxidant nutrients available to protect you from destructive free-radical reactions. Low-fat diets speed the process of degeneration and aging.

Vegetables like broccoli, spinach, and kale are excellent sources of lutein, zeaxanthin, beta-carotene, and other essential nutrients, but if you don't eat them with a source of fat, they will not do as much good, because their beneficial nutrients will not be absorbed. Vitamin A is only available in animal foods. We can convert the beta-carotene in plants into vitamin A, but this can only happen if there is adequate fat in the diet. You can eat fruits and vegetables loaded with antioxidants and other nutrients, but if you don't include fat, you will only absorb a small portion of these vital nutrients. Taking vitamin tablets won't help much because they also require fat to facilitate proper absorption. In this way, a low-fat diet can actually be detrimental.

How much of an effect does fat have on nutrient absorption? Believe it or not, the effect can be highly substantial. In a study conducted at Ohio State University, researchers looked at absorption of three carotenoids (beta-carotene, lycopene, and lutein) in meals that had added fat. The researchers used avocado as the source of the fat.

In the first part of the study, test subjects were given a meal of fat-free salsa and bread. On another day, the same meal was given, but this time avocado was added to the salsa, boosting the fat content of the meal to about 37 percent of calories. Blood levels of the test subjects showed that beta-carotene increased 2.6 times and lycopene 4.4 times. This showed that adding just a little fat to a meal can more than double, triple, or quadruple nutrient absorption.

The second part of the study had the test subjects consume a salad consisting of romaine lettuce, baby spinach, and shredded carrots, with a non-fat dressing. The total fat content of the salad was about 2 percent of calories. After avocado was added, the fat content jumped to 42 percent. The higher-fat salad increased blood levels of lutein 7 times and beta-carotene an incredible 18 times! To put this into perspective, you would need to eat 18 bowls of salad without added oil to equal the amount of beta-carotene you would get from just 1 bowl of salad with a little added fat.

In a similar study, subjects were fed salads using dressings with a different fat content. Salad with non-fat dressing resulted in negligible carotenoid absorption. Low-fat dressing improved nutrient absorption some, but full-fat dressing showed a significant increase. The researchers were surprised not only by how adding fat improved nutrient absorption but also how little is absorbed in the absence of fat.

A number of studies indicate that a diet high in fruits and vegetables, rich sources of essential vitamins and antioxidants, can protect against cancer, heart disease, diabetes, macular degeneration, and other degenerative diseases. Other studies show no benefit to eating fruits and vegetables in regard to preventing degenerative disease. Why the difference in findings? A study conducted in Sweden solved the mystery. This study showed that eating fruits and vegetables did not lower the risk of heart disease *unless* they were eaten with a

118

source of fat, such as full-fat milk, cream, or butter.[18] Eating fruits and vegetables with low-fat milk offered no protective value. We can assume, then, that eating fruits and vegetables won't reduce the risk of any degenerative disease, including eye diseases, unless they are consumed with a source of good fat. Interestingly, in the Swedish study the type of fat that when combined with fruits and vegetables provided the protection against heart disease was saturated fats—from whole milk, cream, and butter.

To get all the nutrients you can from a tomato, carrot, spinach, or any vegetable or low-fat food, add a little fat. Eating vegetables without added fat is, in effect, the same as eating a nutritionally poor meal. Adding a good source of fat in the diet is important in order to gain the most nutrition from your foods. Likewise, taking a multiple vitamin and mineral supplement containing all the best nutrients for eye health will be a waste of time and money unless they are consumed with fat.

Coconut oil appears to be one of the most effective fats, if not the most effective, in improving nutrient absorption. For example, researchers at Auburn University studied the effect of vitamin B_1 (thiamine) deficiency in animals given different types of fats. Vitamin B_1 deficiency leads to a fatal disease called beriberi. The types of oils tested included coconut, olive, flaxseed, cottonseed, butter, lard, and others. When rats were fed a vitamin B-deficient diet, coconut oil was by far more effective than any of the other fats in preventing the disease. Most of the mice in the study began to exhibit symptoms of beriberi after 35-40 days. Those receiving coconut oil however didn't start showing symptoms until after 60 days. A huge difference compared to the other oils. Coconut oil doesn't contain any vitamin B_1, but it made what little of the vitamin that was in the diet more bioavailable, thus preventing or delaying the deficiency disease.

A number of studies have found similar effects. Coconut oil improves the absorption not only of B vitamins but also of vitamins A, D, E, K, beta-carotene, lycopene, lutein, zeaxanthin, and other fat-soluble nutrients.[19] For instance, a recent study compared the absorption of lutein in lutein-deficient mice eating diets containing different types of fat. The fats tested included olive, coconut, peanut, soybean, sunflower, rice bran, corn, palm, and fish oils. Blood levels of lutein were highest in the diets containing olive and coconut oils. Also, lutein accumulation was significantly higher in liver and eye tissue of those animals that had eaten one of these two oils.[20] Another study by a different group of researchers shows that oils rich in saturated fat improve the absorption of lutein and zeaxanthin better than those rich in polyunsaturated or monounsaturated fats.[21]

In comparison to other oils, coconut oil has also shown to improve the absorption of minerals such as calcium, magnesium, and some amino acids—the building blocks for protein.[22] This is one of the reasons why coconut oil or MCTs are added to hospital feeding tube formulas that are given to critically ill patients; coconut oil helps these patients absorb nutrients better and recover more quickly.[23-24]

If you add coconut oil to your meals, you will absorb significantly more vitamins, minerals, and other nutrients than you will if you use soybean, canola, or some other type of oil or no oil at all. Simply adding coconut oil to a meal greatly enhances the overall nutritional value of your food.

This fact has led researchers to investigate the use of coconut oil in the treatment of malnutrition. For example, coconut oil, mixed with a small amount corn oil, was compared with soybean oil for the treatment of malnourished preschool aged children in the Philippines. The study involved 95 children aged 10 to 44 months, who were first-to third-degree malnourished. The children came from a slum area in Manila. They were given one full midday meal and one afternoon snack daily except Sundays for 16 weeks. The food fed to the children was identical in every respect except for the oil. Approximately two-thirds of the oil in their diet came from either the coconut/corn oil mix or soybean oil. The children were allocated to one of the two diets at random: 47 children received the coconut oil diet, and 48 children the soybean oil diet.

The children were weighed every two weeks and examined by a pediatrician once a week. At the start of the study the ages, initial weight, and degree of malnutrition of the two groups as a whole were essentially identical.

After the 16 weeks, results showed that the coconut oil diet produced significantly faster weight gain and improvement in nutritional status compared to the soybean oil diet. A mean gain of 5.57 pounds, due to improved growth and nutritional status, was recorded after four months for the coconut oil group, almost twice as much as the weight gain of the soybean oil groups of 3.27 pounds.

Not only does coconut oil improve absorption of most vitamins and minerals, but it also helps preserve antioxidants. Diets high in polyunsaturated oils (including fish oils) drain the body's antioxidant reserves. Coconut oil does the opposite, it acts like a protective antioxidant, preventing lipid peroxidation and, thus, preserving available antioxidants.[25-26] Replacing polyunsaturated vegetable oils in food preparation with coconut oil can significantly improve your antioxidant and nutrient status, thereby reducing the risks of developing free-radical associated degenerative diseases.

Vitamin and mineral absorption improves so much with the addition of fat that if you eat an adequate amount of fresh fruits and vegetables combined with good sources of fat—primarily coconut and red palm—you likely will not even need to add any supplements to your diet.

AN EGG A DAY MAY KEEP THE EYE DOCTOR AWAY

If you are looking for foods that are highly nutritious, contain a balanced source of protein, fat, vitamins, and minerals necessary for both a healthy body and healthy eyes, eggs would have to be at the top of the list. For many years eggs have been shunned by the diet police because of their high cholesterol content. Egg whites, without the yolks, have become a common food item for people who are trying to cut back on their fat and cholesterol intake in the hopes of reducing their risk of heart disease. Although a large egg yolk contains 210 mg of cholesterol, studies repeatedly show that they do not have a negative impact on blood cholesterol levels, nor do they increase the risk of heart disease.

Eggs tend to raise HDL cholesterol, the so-called "good" cholesterol that is believed to protect against heart disease. The higher your HDL cholesterol, the better. Studies at the University of Connecticut have shown that eating three eggs a day for 30 days increased total cholesterol slightly, but that was due primarily to an increase in HDL cholesterol. The ratio between HDL and LDL (the so-called "bad" cholesterol), which is universally recognized as a much better indicator of heart disease risk than total cholesterol, did not change. Eating three eggs a day had no detrimental effect on cholesterol levels and did not increase heart disease risk.

In a study by researchers at Harvard in 1999, of nearly 120,000 men and women, no association was found between egg consumption and heart disease. Since then, many studies have similarly vindicated eggs, including a Japanese study published in the *British Journal of Nutrition* in 2006, which involved more than 90,000 middle-aged people, and a study in 2007 from the University of Medicine and Dentistry of New Jersey. Both of these studies found no link between frequent egg consumption and heart disease. In light of these findings, nutritionists have welcomed eggs back into what they consider a healthy diet.

Egg yolks, organ meats, shellfish, and whole-fat dairy products are good sources of dietary cholesterol, but they don't have much effect on blood cholesterol. About 80 percent of the cholesterol in our blood is produced in our own bodies by our liver and is not a reflection of the cholesterol in our diet. One of the biggest problems with giving up eggs is that people turn to other breakfast foods like bagels, cold cereal, pastries, and muffins. These are loaded with unhealthy sugar and refined grains, which increase blood cholesterol levels far more than eggs ever could.

Ironically, eggs may help prevent heart disease because of the beneficial nutrients they contain. Here are some interesting and little-known facts about eggs:

• Egg yolks are a rich source of lutein and zeaxanthin, which can help keep eyes healthy and reduce risk of age-related degenerative disease. Lutein and zeaxanthin from eggs are better absorbed by the body than those from spinach or supplements. A study in the *Journal of Nutrition* in 2006 found that women who ate six eggs a week for 12 weeks had increased macular pigment, which protects the retina from the damaging effects of high-energy light.

• One large egg contains 6 grams of high-quality protein (in both the yolk and the white). The yolk is also a source of vitamin A, the B vitamins (including riboflavin and folate), zinc, and other nutrients.

• Egg yolks provide choline, an essential nutrient especially important for fetal brain development. Researchers have also identified other compounds in eggs that may have anti-cancer, anti-hypertensive, immune-boosting, and antioxidant properties.

• Free-range chickens that have access to growing grass, convert the plant based omega-3s in these plants to the more biologically active DHA form. They also have a higher lutein and zeaxanthin content than conventionally produced eggs.

• Brown eggs are not more nutritious than white. Different breeds of chickens simply lay eggs with different shell colors, even blue and green. Yolk color depends on what the chicken ate: wheat and barley produce a light yolk; corn a medium yellow yolk; and marigold petals a deep yellow. Darker yellow or orange-yellow yolk indicates a higher lutein and zeaxanthin content. This is why organic eggs often have darker yolks.

• Eggs help with weight management by improving satiety, due in part to their fat and protein content. In a study of overweight women, reported in the *Journal of the American College of Nutrition* in 2005, those who ate two eggs for breakfast felt fuller afterward and ate significantly fewer calories at lunch than women who consumed a bagel-based breakfast with the same number of calories.

Making whole eggs or egg yolks a part of your regular diet may help keep age-related macular degeneration and other degenerative eye disorders at bay. Two studies published in the *Journal of Nutrition*

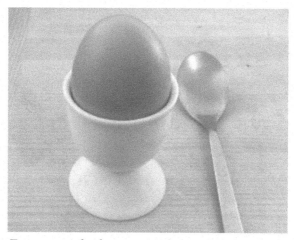

Eggs provide the eyes with good nutrition.

suggest that eating an egg a day can boost blood and eye levels of lutein and zeaxanthin and reduce the risk of AMD.

In the first study, investigators measured blood levels of lutein and zeaxanthin in volunteers over the age of 60 after eating one egg or an egg substitute daily for five weeks. In comparison to the group who ate egg substitute, eating one egg daily increased lutein and zeaxanthin levels by 26 to 38 percent. The researchers also reported that adding the eggs into the subject's diets had no effect on cholesterol or triglyceride levels.[27]

In the second study, investigators also looked at the effect of egg consumption on blood levels of lutein and zeaxanthin, as well as macular pigment optical density (MOPD), a yellow pigment in the macula made of those carotenoids. The density of the pigment indicates how much lutein and zeaxanthin are absorbed from the bloodstream and incorporated into the eyes, where they are needed to protect against AMD. Volunteers ate 6 eggs a week for 12 weeks. MOPD increased significantly with egg consumption in comparison to the placebo group, who did not eat the eggs. Interestingly, total cholesterol and triglyceride levels of the egg consumers remained unchanged but increased in the placebo group.[28]

8

The Miracle of Ketones

CALORIE RESTRICTION

On September 26, 1991, eight scientists, four men and four women, embarked on a two-year mission designed to explore the possibility of living and colonizing distant moons and planets. The crew was to remain in the Biosphere 2 for the entire two years, living off food they produced themselves and breathing the air produced by the plants that they brought with them. The Biosphere 2 was not a space station or rocket ship, but an enclosed, airtight structure built at the base of the Santa Catalina Mountains in Arizona.

The Biosphere 2 enclosed an area the size of two and a half football fields. It was divided into various environmental zones that included a rainforest, mini-ocean with a coral reef, mangrove wetlands, a 2,500 square-meter agricultural area for raising crops, and a human habitat and research station. Heating and cooling water circulated through independent piping systems and passive solar input through glass space frame panels covering most of the facility.

Once the scientists entered the structure, the door was sealed and they were to remain inside for the full two years of the experiment. Trouble struck the crew early on when their food crops were devastated by disease. Food had to be severely rationed for most of the rest of the experiment. The health of the participants was monitored by Roy Walford, MD, a professor of pathology at UCLA and a member of the crew.

Interestingly, the lack of food did not harm the crew. In fact, their health dramatically improved during their forced dietary restriction. Within six months, average weight decreased by 26 pounds in the men, 15 pounds in the women. Blood pressure levels dropped from an average of 110/75 to 90/58, and memory, mood, and energy levels also improved. Risk factors associated with heart disease, diabetes, cancer, and other degenerative conditions all fell to optimal levels. Essentially, they became physically and mentally younger and healthier.

Dr. Walford was so impressed by the dramatic positive changes in the participants' health that he began researching the effects of calorie restriction on health and longevity and wrote many bestselling books on the topic.

Dr. Walford, however, wasn't the first to notice improvement in health in correlation with a decrease in food consumption. As early as 1915 it was reported that restricting the food intake of rodents resulted in a considerable increase in their maximum lifespan. This phenomenon was explored in more detail in the 1930s by C.M. McCay and colleagues at Cornell University. McCay learned that underfed rodents were generally healthier and lived up to 40 percent longer than their well-fed counterparts. Over the years, these results have been duplicated in fruit flies, worms, fish, monkeys, and other animals.

Calorie restriction is often referred to as an "anti-aging diet" because it slows the aging process and extends lifespan. It also provides protection against numerous degenerative diseases that tend to shorten life. For example, one published report shows that breast cancer incidence fell from 40 percent in fully fed animals to only 2 percent in calorie-restricted animals; lung cancer fell from 60 to 30 percent; liver cancer fell from 64 to 0 percent; leukemia from 65 to 10 percent; kidney disease from 100 to 36 percent; and cardiovascular disease fell from 63 to 17 percent.[1]

Other conditions that are delayed or avoided by calorie restriction include arthritis, diabetes, atherosclerosis, Alzheimer's, Parkinson's, Huntington's, and virtually all age-related degenerative diseases.[2-3]

In animal studies, 40 to 50 percent calorie restriction has produced the greatest extension in lifespan. In humans, restricting calories this much is too difficult to maintain. A 25 percent restriction is more doable. A normal 2,000 calorie diet would be reduced to 1,500 calories. Even still, it takes a great deal of willpower to maintain this level of restriction for life. At this level, human studies have reported improvement in various measures of health status, similar to those seen in animal studies. A change in maximum lifespan has not yet been determined because the studies have not gone on long enough.

Since the total amount of food is decreased, what is eaten must be nutrient dense, and empty calories like those found in junk foods must be avoided. Eating empty calories on a restricted diet will lead to malnutrition. This is why semi-starved populations in certain parts of the world don't live longer—they are calorie restricted and malnourished.

Calorie restriction can be accomplished in a number of ways. The most obvious is to simply reduce the number of calories consumed each day. Another method is to reduce the number of days on which food is allowed. Food can be eaten every other day or just three or four days a week. This is called intermittent fasting. The health benefits are still there even when there is no restriction on calorie intake on the days when food is eaten. Another form of intermittent fasting is to limit eating to an 8 hour period of time each day. In this case, a person would fast for 16 hours out of every 24. In such a case, eating may be restricted to ten a.m. to six p.m. with no limit on the amount eaten during that time period.

There are many reasons why reducing total calorie intake or fasting periodically produces such remarkable health benefits. Calorie restriction is known to increase DNA repair, decrease oxidative damage, increase the body's own antioxidant defense system, lower blood pressure and inflammation, improve glucose metabolism and insulin sensitivity, delay age-related immunological decline, and it is associated with less glycation; all of these undoubtedly play a part in the improved health and longevity.

One of the most important effects of calorie restriction in regard to brain and nerve health is the activation of a special group of protective proteins known as neurotrophic factors. One type in particular, brain-derived neurotrophic factors (BDNF), plays a key role in regulating survival, growth, and maintenance of neurons, and is important for learning and memory. BDNF regulate the neurotransmitters (e.g., dopamine, glutamate) that carry chemical signals, which allow neurons to communicate with each other. They protect neurons from the detrimental effects of various toxins and stressors that can harm brain and nerve tissue.[4-5] BDNF help to support the survival of existing neurons and encourage the growth and differentiation of new neurons. Although the majority of neurons in the human brain are formed before birth, parts of the adult brain retain the ability to grow new neurons from neural stem cells in a process known as neurogenesis. Neurotrophic factors help stimulate and control neurogenesis. BDNF also play a significant role in the maintenance of brain cell function throughout an individual's lifetime.

Calorie restriction can have a profound effect on preserving eye health. As we age, subtle changes gradually occur in the visual system. Lifelong exposure to free radicals takes its toll on the lens, retina, and other tissues. Oxidative stress caused by exposure to excessive free radicals is generally most noticeable in the clouding of the lens, leading to cataracts. Calorie restriction reduces the amount of free radicals generated in the eye from normal metabolic processes. Several animal studies have shown the beneficial effects in retarding cataract formation.[6-8] In animal studies, a reduction of 40 percent of calories delays the onset, formation, progression, and accumulation of cataracts. Even a reduction of 20 percent of calories has shown to be beneficial.

Photoreceptors in the retina are the most vulnerable cells in the eye when it comes to age-related deterioration. Retinal cell density and thickness of the inner retina and macula normally decline gradually with age. Over the course of your lifetime, as much as 30 percent of your rod cells are lost. Of the three cone cells, the blue-sensitive ones are the least numerous and the most likely to die from repeated exposure to light. Calorie restriction exhibits a neuroprotective effect on the aging retina and reduces age-related photoreceptor cell death.[9] In lab animals, a 40 percent reduction in caloric intake, in comparison to no reduction, has shown to significantly reduce retinal cell loss.[10]

Retinal pigment cells are also highly vulnerable to degeneration with age. The accumulation of a substance called lipofuscin in and around retinal pigment cells leads to functional loss of the retina. Lipofuscin is an aggregate of yellow-brown granules composed of oxidized unsaturated fatty acids and protein. It is believed to be caused by cell membrane damage. Lipofuscin, which is a byproduct of free radicals, also generates free radicals and must be removed to avoid further damage. Retinal pigment cells absorb lipofuscin and attempt to break it down and discard it. Over time, however, lipofuscin can accumulate, promoting degeneration of the retina. Lipofuscin accumulation is a major risk factor implicated in age-related macular degeneration as well as Stargardt disease (juvenile macular degeneration). Lipofuscin is produced in other tissues and is found in the brains of those with Alzheimer's, Parkinson's, amyotrophic lateral sclerosis (ALS), and other degenerative diseases.

The accumulation of lipofuscin appears to be a universal feature of the aging process. In mammals, lipofuscin content of the retinal pigment cells increases progressively with age. Dietary restriction has shown to substantially reduce the rate of lipofuscin accumulation in the retina.[11]

Aging leads to an inherent loss of retinal ganglion cells, which come together to form the optic nerve (see diagram on page 18). With age, these cells, as well as others, become more susceptible to harm and degenerate faster when exposed to damaging stressful conditions such as free radicals, sunlight, poor blood supply, inflammation, increased intraocular pressure, etc.

Increased intraocular pressure, caused by defects in the ocular drainage system, is the main risk factor for glaucoma. Elevated pressure can lead to optic nerve damage and subsequent loss of vision. Calorie restriction prevents the defect that causes the blockage in the ocular drainage system, thus maintaining normal intraocular pressure and preserving the optic nerve.[12-13]

Restricting the flow of blood and oxygen to cells will cause their death. When this happens in the brain, it leads to a stroke. In the laboratory setting, researchers temporarily cut off blood flow to the retina to examine its effects. When old rats that have been on a calorie-restricted diet are subjected to this procedure, they experience significantly less loss of retinal ganglion cells in comparison to normally fed rats of similar age or even younger rats that tend to endure stress better than aged rats.[14]

Calorie restriction has proven to be protective against a wide range of neurological conditions, many of which affect eyesight. It is also known to increase numbers of newly generated neural cells in the adult brain, suggesting that this dietary manipulation can increase the brain's capacity for plasticity and self-repair.[15] This leads to the possibility that certain degenerative eye diseases may be preventable and even reversible, at least to some extent.

EXERCISE STRENGTHENS THE BRAIN AND EYES

"If exercise could be packaged in pill form, it would immediately become the number-one anti-aging medicine, as well as the world's most prescribed pill," says Dr. Robert Butler of the International Longevity Center at Manhattan's Mount Sinai Hospital. Exercise improves blood pressure, balances blood sugar and insulin levels, protects against heart disease, improves brain and nerve function, and reduces risk of macular degeneration and other age-related eye disorders. In fact, many of the same benefits associated with calorie restriction are also gained by exercise. The added benefit of exercise is that it also tones the muscles, strengthens the bones, and increases energy levels.

Just as exercise can bulk up the muscles, it can also bulk up the brain—literally! Regular exercise stimulates brain cell growth and repair, just as it does for the muscles. Exercise tones the brain and slows the aging process.

As neurons age and die, the brain shrinks, and cognitive ability declines. Most people assume that brain shrinkage begins when we reach middle age or later. But actually, shrinkage begins as early as your 30s and normally progresses at a rate of about 0.5 to 1 percent a year.

According to a study by Dr. Arthur Kramer and colleagues at the University of Illinois-Urbana, the rate at which the brain ages (i.e., shrinks) can be dramatically slowed with just three hours of aerobic exercise a week. Kramer divided a group of 59 adults, aged 60 to 79 years, into two groups and monitored them for six months. One group participated in 1 hour of aerobics three times a week, at a level of 60 to 70 percent of their maximum heart rate. The other group spent 1 hour three times a week doing stretching and toning exercises. Three-dimensional MRI scans of the participants' brains were taken at the beginning and end of the study period. This allowed the researchers to visually compare the before and after pictures of the participants' brains. Kramer found that after only six months, the participants who exercised aerobically had the brain volume of people three years younger. Not only did aerobic exercise prevent brain shrinkage, but it also stimulated neuron growth, and the exercisers actually regained lost brain mass. Most of the growth occurred in the frontal lobe of the brain, which is involved in memory and reasoning. There was no improvement in the brains of those who did only toning and stretching exercises.[16]

Why was there such remarkable improvement? Exercise improves brain health, in part by improving circulation. More blood, which carries oxygen and nutrients, is brought in to feed and nourish the brain. Exercise reduces insulin resistance and improves glucose metabolism, allowing the brain to function better. In addition, exercise stimulates the activation of special neuroprotective proteins such as BDNF and insulin-like growth factor 1 (IGF-1), both of which defend the brain against oxidative stress and promote neuron growth and repair.

Not only does exercise slow the normal aging process, but it also protects against neurodegenerative diseases such as Alzheimer's and Parkinson's. Dr. E.B. Larson and colleagues at the Center for Health Studies in Seattle, Washington, found that persons 65 years of age and older who exercised three or more times per week, experienced a much lower rate of Alzheimer's disease than those who exercised less or not at all.[17]

In another study, brisk walking improved memory in elderly people who were at high risk of developing Alzheimer's. The study involved 138 men aged 50 years and older, all of whom reported memory problems but had not yet met the criteria for dementia diagnosis. The participants were divided into two groups. One began a 24-week exercise program of walking for 50 minutes three days per week, while the other group continued at their normal activity level. After 24 weeks, participants in the exercise group scored better on memory assessments and cognitive tests and lower on dementia ratings. Those in the control group, on the other hand, showed a decline, as would be expected as part of the normal process of aging and continued brain shrinkage. The positive effects of the exercise were still evident 18 months later.[18] The researchers stated that the effects of exercise were better than those seen with drugs approved to aid mental function in Alzheimer's disease.

Even in Alzheimer's patients, for whom brain shrinkage can be severe, exercise improves brain volume. The area of the brain most involved in storing and retrieving memory—the hippocampus—is protected from shrinkage.[19]

Researchers at St. Jude Children's Research Hospital in Memphis, Tennessee demonstrated that exercise increases the brain's capacity for self-repair. They showed that neurotoxic drugs which damage areas of the brain that control movement and induce Parkinson's disease were rendered completely harmless by regular exercise.[20]

Studies such as those described above suggest that exercise not only slows the natural aging process but can potentially provide protection against a variety of neurodegenerative conditions. In essence, exercise acts as an antidote against neurodegeneration.

Exercise also protects the retina from age-related degeneration. In 2009, a study of more than 40,000 middle-aged distance runners found that those who covered the most miles had the least likelihood of developing macular degeneration.[21] The study, however, did not compare runners to non-runners and did not try to explain how exercise protected the retina.

Researchers at Emory University in Atlanta and the Atlanta Veterans Administration Medical Center took up those questions.[22] Their curiosity was piqued by animal research that was being done at the Veterans Administration. They found that exercise increased the level of growth factors in the bloodstream and brain of animals, in particular BDNF, which is known to promote the regeneration and health of neurons. The retina also contains neurons, so the researchers wondered whether exercise might raise levels of BDNF there as well, potentially affecting retinal health and vision.

To test that idea, the researchers placed a group of mice on treadmills for an hour a day. Another group of mice were allowed to remain sedentary throughout the day. After two weeks, half the mice in each group were exposed to an intensely bright light for four hours, while the other animals stayed in dimly lit cages. This light exposure is a widely used and accepted means of inducing retinal degeneration in animals. It obviously doesn't precisely mimic the slowly progressing disease in humans, but it does cause a comparable, time-compressed loss of retinal neurons.

The mice then returned to their former routines, either running or not running, for another two weeks, after which the scientists measured the number of neurons in each animal's eyes. The unexercised mice exposed to the bright light had begun to experience severe retinal degeneration; almost 75 percent of the retinal photoreceptors had died. The mice that had exercised before being exposed to the light retained about twice as many functional photoreceptors as the sedentary animals; in addition, those cells were more responsive to normal light than the surviving retinal neurons in the unexercised mice. Exercise, it seems, made the running rodents' retinas more resilient.

In addition, the researchers had other mice run or sit around for two weeks, then measured levels of BDNF in their eyes and bloodstreams. The runners had far more. When the scientists injected other mice with a chemical that blocks the uptake of the growth factor before allowing them to run and exposing them to the bright light, their eyes deteriorated as badly as the sedentary rodents. When the mice could not utilize BDNF, exercise did not protect their eyes. These experiments demonstrate that exercise protects vision by increasing the level of BDNF in the retina.

Many studies have shown a clear benefit to brain and eye health with aerobic exercise, which involves continuous, vigorous movement and includes activities such as jogging, swimming laps, or hiking. Weightlifting, a non-aerobic exercise, is less beneficial as far as eye health is concerned. Human studies have consistently shown that the longer the duration or more vigorous the aerobic exercise, the greater the effect on increasing levels of BDNF.[23-25]

Moderate to heavy intensity exercise is needed to produce a significant increase in BDNF.[26] In other words, a leisurely 30 minute walk won't have too much effect on BDNF, while a brisk 30 minute walk will. The higher the intensity, the greater the effect. A study of active runners found that the risk of age-related retinal degeneration is decreased by 10 percent for every kilometer/day increment in running distance.[27]

THE KETOGENIC DIET

Years ago it was discovered that fasting, consuming nothing but water, can have a pronounced therapeutic effect on the body.

In contrast to intermittent fasting where short periods of fasting are separated by periods of eating, fasting therapy consists of total abstinence from food and drink, except water, for several days or weeks at a time. In the early 1900s doctors often used fasting therapy to treat many chronic health problems such as arthritis, dermatitis, digestive disturbances, and psychiatric disorders. One of the conditions that responded exceptionally well to fasting therapy was epilepsy, a neurological disorder characterized by abnormal electrical activity in the brain that leads to sudden recurrent seizures. These episodes can vary from a simple blank, frozen stare that may last just a few seconds to violent, uncontrollable thrashing of the arms and legs and loss of consciousness. Epileptics can suffer with as many as 100 or more seizures a day. Placing epileptic patient's on a water only fast for 14 to 30 days brought about a remarkable decrease in seizures, with long-lasting results. As a result of fasting therapy, most epileptic patients experience a dramatic reduction in seizures, and some become totally seizure-free. The effects may last for months, years, or even for life.

Doctors noticed that the longer they kept a patient on a fast, the better the outcome. However, there is a limit to how long a person can remain on a fast consuming nothing but water. In the early 1920s doctors began looking into developing a diet that could mimic the therapeutic effects of fasting yet allow enough nutrients to support good health. The result was the ketogenic diet.

The ketogenic diet consists of eating a high proportion of fat, a moderate amount of protein, just a little carbohydrate, and absolutely no sugar. Normally, about 55 to 60 percent of our daily calories comes from carbohydrates. In the classic ketogenic diet, carbohydrate is reduced to just 2 to 3 percent of total calories consumed. In adults who consume 2,000 calories daily, this equates to about 10 to 15 grams per day. Since calories from carbohydrate are reduced so dramatically, another source of calories is necessary to make up the difference. In the ketogenic diet, these calories come from fat, which provides the basic building blocks for ketones. Fat comprises around 86 to 90 percent of daily calories. Protein makes up the rest (about 8 percent of total calories). The ketogenic diet is not high in protein. It contains an adequate amount of protein to maintain good health. The ketogenic diet can best be described as a high-fat, adequate-protein, very low-carb diet.

Under normal conditions, our bodies burn glucose for energy. We get glucose primarily from carbohydrates in our foods. During fasting, when no carbohydrates are consumed, fat in our bodies is pulled out of storage and fatty acids are released into the bloodstream to supply the necessary energy. Some of this fat is converted by the liver into water-soluble compounds (beta-hydroxybutyrate, acetoacetate, and acetone), collectively known as ketone bodies, or ketones. Ketones are used by the cells as an alternative form of energy. During a fast, blood ketones rise, and a person is said to be in ketosis. Ketosis can also be achieved by limiting the amount of carbohydrate in the diet. A low-carb diet can bring about a state of ketosis. In 1921, Dr. Russel Wilder of the Mayo Clinic coined the term "ketogenic diet" to describe a diet that produces a high level of ketones in the blood through the consumption of a high-fat, low-carbohydrate diet. He was the first to use the ketogenic diet as a treatment for epilepsy.

The ketogenic diet has proven incredibly successful in treating even the most severe forms of epilepsy. Not only does it significantly reduce the number of seizures, but in many cases, it can also bring about a complete cure. The diet is used primarily for children who continue with the treatment for about two years. Dietary restrictions are then gradually relaxed until the patient can eat a normal diet.

Since the ketogenic diet proved to be useful in correcting the brain defects associated with epilepsy, researchers began to test it on other brain and nerve disorders. Evidence from animal studies and human clinical studies show that the ketogenic diet can bring improvement to a broad range of neurodegenerative conditions including narcolepsy (a sleep disorder characterized by sudden, uncontrollable urges to sleep), depression, migraine headaches, Alzheimer's, Parkinson's, Huntington's, ALS, autism, traumatic brain injury, and stroke. The ketogenic diet has also been associated with improvement in cognitive function.[28-37]

In tissue cultures, ketone bodies have been shown to increase the survival of motor neurons—the neurons that control movement. This is important for those with ALS, a neurodegenerative disorder that affects motor neurons and is characterized by progressive muscle weakness and paralysis and eventually leads to death.

In a mouse model of ALS, researchers fed a ketogenic diet to mice that were genetically modified to develop the disease. Physical strength and performance in these mice was preserved in comparison to mice fed a standard diet. On autopsy, it was found that the ketogenic-fed mice had significantly higher numbers of surviving motor neurons than the control mice.

Huntington's disease is an inherited condition that causes the progressive degeneration of neurons in the brain. The disease usually results in movement, cognitive, and psychiatric disorders. The mice used to study Huntington's disease are bred to have the modified huntingtin gene. Dietary intervention that increases blood ketones has shown to delay the onset of the disease and extend the lives of the mice up to 15 percent longer. In humans, that would equate to an additional 10 to 12 years.

Tissue cultures from dopaminergic and hippocampal cells of the brain (areas affected by Parkinson's and Alzheimer's disease) are also protected by ketones.[38] MPTP, a neurotoxic drug that causes the destruction of dopamine neurons, is administered to animals to mimic Parkinson's disease. Ketones, however, protect the dopamine neurons in these animals from the harmful effects of MPTP, allowing them to maintain energy production and function.[39]

Ketones not only stop neurodegeneration, but they can restore lost function as well. This was demonstrated in a clinical study with Parkinson's patients by Dr. Theodore VanItallie and colleagues at Columbia University College of Physicians and Surgeons. "Ketones are a high-energy fuel that nourish the brain," says Dr. VanItallie. The study involved five Parkinson's patients who were put on a ketogenic diet for 28 days. All of the participants' tremors, stiffness, balance, and ability to walk improved, on average, by a remarkable 43 percent.[40]

The participants maintained a classic ketogenic diet consisting of about 90 percent fat. Initially, seven subjects volunteered for the study, but one dropped out the first week because the diet was too difficult to maintain and the other dropped out for personal reasons. Three of the five participants who completed the study adhered faithfully to the prescribed menu. The other two participants did not adhere to the diet as strictly but still achieved and maintained ketosis throughout the study. Each participant was evaluated using the Unified Parkinson's Disease Rating Scale at the beginning and end of the study. When the scores were compared, every subject showed marked improvement. Interestingly, the two participants who were not as strict with the diet and had slightly lower blood ketone levels improved the most, one by 46 percent and the other by 81. This indicates that a classic ketogenic diet may not be necessary, and a less restrictive diet, such as a modified low-carb diet, may be just as or even more effective.

In animal studies, ketones significantly reduce the amount of amyloid plaque that develops in Alzheimer's disease.[41-42] In dog models of the disease, ketones improve daytime activity, increase performance on visual-spatial memory tasks, increase probability of learning tasks, have superior performance on motor learning tasks, and increase performance in short-term memory.[43] A number of studies show that ketones protect the brain from injury and promote rapid healing after an injury.[44-46]

Ketones also stimulate the production and activity of neurotrophic factors, including BDNF, which are critical to the health and survival of neurons.[47] Almost all clinical studies using drugs as a means to protect the retina, optic nerve, and other components of the eye have failed. BDNF, however, shows promise. Since ketones increase the levels of BDNF in the retina, the ketogenic diet has been proposed as a means to protect against glaucoma and other retinal degenerative diseases.[48]

Ketones can be utilized by nearly every cell and organ in the body.[49] Almost every disease state, whether in the brain or elsewhere, involves runaway inflammation and poor oxygen and glucose utilization. Ketones improve oxygen utilization and calms inflammation, thereby potentially providing protection against a large number of disease conditions.

In addition to restoring brain health, the ketogenic diet improves many other aspects of health as well. It has shown to reduce high blood pressure, aid in the loss of excess body fat, improve concentration, stabilize and moderate blood sugar and insulin levels, improve blood cholesterol and triglyceride levels, calm inflammation, and reduce risk of cancer, among other things. In essence, a ketogenic diet can bring about the same metabolic improvements seen in calorie restriction and exercise.

THE COMMON DENOMINATOR

Calorie restriction in its various forms, moderate to heavy exercise, and eating a low-carb ketogenic diet are all known to produce similar positive effects on both overall and neurological health. Each of these approaches share some important metabolic effects, including increased burning of fat in place of glucose, increased production and utilization of ketones, and reduced blood glucose levels.

Degenerative disease is often associated with elevated levels of glucose, insulin, and triglycerides. People who live long lives in relatively good health have lower blood glucose, insulin, and serum triglycerides. Researchers at Duke University and the University of Arizona have shown that the fundamental mechanism by which calorie restriction and intermittent fasting improve health and prolong life is by an alternation in these metabolic parameters. Using a ketogenic diet, the researchers were able to duplicate the metabolic effects of calorie restriction completely and independently of caloric intake. The diet is based on the premise that by shifting much of the body's dependence on energy from glucose to fat, many of the same physiologic changes seen in calorie-restricted animals will also be seen in individuals following such a diet.[50]

Patients in the study were told to eat when they were hungry. Calories were not explicitly restricted; calorie intake was determined solely by appetite. Protein intake was limited to approximately 1.0 g/kg lean body mass per day. As a result, most patients were instructed to eat from 50 to 80 grams of protein per day. Only non-starchy, fibrous vegetables were allowed. Though not explicitly stated, the general dietary intake as percent of daily caloric intake for most participants ended up to be approximately 20 percent carbohydrate, 20 percent protein, and 60 percent fat.

The study lasted for three months. During this time patients lost on average, 7 pounds (3 kg) of excess body weight, even though they were not dieting and ate as much as they wanted. They showed a significant reduction in blood pressure, an average drop of over 10 mmHg. Blood insulin and fasting glucose significantly decreased. Insulin sensitivity improved. In addition, despite the increased intake of fat, they experienced a significant decrease in triglyceride levels. Their triglyceride/HDL ratios decreased on average, from 5.1 to 2.6, which is very significant, since triglyceride/HDL ratio is considered one of the most accurate indicators of heart disease risk.[51] A ratio of 4.0 or greater indicates high risk. The patients' beginning average of 5.1 was much too high, but by the end of the study the average ratio dropped to a much safer 2.6. A ratio of 2.0 is considered ideal, so within just three months on a high-fat, low-carb diet, they went from being at very high risk of heart disease to low risk, as well as lowering their risk of diabetes and a multitude of other health problems, thus avoiding or delaying diseases that would otherwise shorten their lives.

Longevity studies using calorie restriction examine the same metabolic parameters measured in this study. This and other studies demonstrate clearly that high-fat, low-carbohydrate diets produce the same physiological effects as calorie restriction, only without all the drawbacks like constant hunger, low energy, depressed metabolism, and disturbed hormone balance.

Simply put, the ketogenic diet is more effective than calorie-restricted diets. In fact, studies show that a low-carb, high-fat diet produces better results on metabolic parameters than calorie restriction. One study did a direct comparison of the two diets. Investigators compared a low-carb, high-fat ketogenic diet to a calorie-restricted diet over a 24-week period in patients with obesity and type 2 diabetes. The low-carb diet was restricted to 20 grams or less of carbohydrate a day, with no explicit limitation on total calorie intake. The calorie-restricted diet was 500 calories per day lower than normal, about a 25 percent reduction. Both diets led to improvements in metabolic parameters.

Metabolic measurements included fasting glucose, blood triglyceride levels, HDL (good) cholesterol levels, total cholesterol/HDL cholesterol ratio, triglyceride/HDL cholesterol ratio, blood pressure, waist circumference, body weight, and body mass index. In every case, the measurements of the low-carb group exceeded those of the calorie-restricted group. It is interesting that the low-carb group consumed more calories than the calorie-restricted group, yet they lost more weight and more inches around the waist. This is apparently a result of superior metabolic control and improved insulin sensitivity in the low-carb group. In diabetic patients taking insulin, the effects were often dramatic. For example, participants taking 40 to 90 units of insulin before the study were able to eliminate their insulin use while also improving glycemic control. Over 95 percent of the participants in the low-carb group were able to reduce or completely eliminate their medications (insulin, metformin, pioglitazone, glimiperide) by the end of the study. The results of this study are in agreement with a number of other studies that have evaluated the metabolic effects of low-carb, high-fat diets.[52-56]

The major conclusion that can be made from these studies is that the reason why calorie restriction protects against degenerative disease and prolongs life is not due to the reduction in calories; rather, it is due to the reduction in carbohydrates. A low-carb diet that does not restrict calories produces better changes in metabolic parameters without the adverse side effects associated with calorie restriction. The true anti-aging diet, therefore, is one that supplies enough protein to meet the body's needs, with fat replacing much of the carbohydrate so as to maintain adequate calorie consumption. Basically, this is a low-carb diet with no restriction on fat consumption. This type of diet has proven to improve insulin sensitivity and glucose metabolism and reduce inflammation, glycation, and free-radical generation, thereby protecting the brain and eyes from degenerative disease.[57]

THE THERAPEUTIC EFFECTS OF KETONES

Another shared characteristic between calorie restriction in its many forms and the ketogenic diet is the increase in ketone production. This is very important.

Like a car, our cells need fuel to run. Glucose is like the gasoline you put in your car. It is the primary source of energy used by all the cells in the body. We get glucose primarily from the carbohydrate in our foods. When food is not eaten for a time, such as between meals, during sleep, or when fasting, blood glucose levels fall. However, our cells demand a continual supply of energy 24 hours a day. To maintain this energy, stored body fat is mobilized and fatty acids are released. Our cells use fatty acids just like they do glucose to produce energy. In this manner, our cells always have access to either glucose or fatty acids. While this process works well for the body, it doesn't work for the brain.

Fatty acids cannot cross the blood-brain barrier, so the brain cannot use them to satisfy its energy needs. When blood glucose levels begin to fall, the brain needs an alternative source of energy.

This alternative fuel source comes in the form of ketones. Ketones are a special type of high-energy fuel produced in the liver specifically to nourish the brain. Almost all the cells in the body can use ketones for energy, but they are made specifically to feed the brain. Between meals, when blood glucose levels decline, the liver starts producing ketones and blood ketone levels increase. After a meal, as glucose levels rise, the liver stops producing ketones, and blood ketone levels decline. This way, the brain has a continual supply of energy from either glucose or ketones.

The metabolic demands of the retina are very high. Although glucose is thought to be the primary source of energy for the retina, ketone bodies also play an important role.[58] Ketones are referred to as "superfuel" for the brain, since they provide more energy than what can be derived from glucose. They are something like a high-performance gasoline for your car, providing more power and better mileage, with less wear on the engine. Ketones have a similar effect on the brain and eyes: improved performance and function with less wear and tear.

Ketones are absolutely essential for brain health and survival. The brain requires a great deal of energy. In fact, the nervous system consumes about two-thirds of the total glucose normally used each day. When the body is at rest, the brain itself uses about one-fifth of all the body's energy. Blood glucose levels fluctuate throughout the day and night, and ketones are necessary when blood glucose levels decline. Without ketones, the brain cells would starve and degenerate.

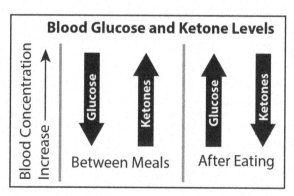

Blood glucose and ketone levels rise and fall according to our eating patterns and the types of food in our diet.

Dead and dying brain cells cause inflammation and increase free-radical formation, but ketones maintain energy levels and prevent this from happening.

Most neurological disorders (Alzheimer's, Parkinson's, glaucoma, macular degeneration, diabetic retinopathy, etc.) are almost always accompanied by oxidative stress and chronic inflammation. Inflammation causes insulin resistance. Chronic inflammation in the brain leads to chronic insulin resistance in the brain. When the brain is insulin resistant, it is unable to effectively absorb glucose. Brain cells begin to die, causing more inflammation, releasing more free radicals, and intensifying insulin resistance. Unlike glucose, ketones are not affected by insulin resistance. They bypass the defect in glucose metabolism and provide the brain cells with the energy they need to maintain proper function.

The human brain is one of the most metabolically active organs in the body, and therefore, needs a high amount of oxygen. The adult brain accounts for only 2 percent of the body's total mass, yet consumes about 20 percent of the oxygen inhaled. This amount of oxygen needs to be supplied to the brain continually. If we are prevented from breathing for even a few minutes we will die of suffocation. Likewise, if the brain's supply of oxygen is cut off or decreased, the brain will die of suffocation within minutes. This is exactly what happens during a stroke. If a blood vessel that feeds the brain becomes clogged or ruptures, disrupting normal blood flow, brain cells cannot get the oxygen they need, and they begin to suffocate and die.

Ketones decrease the brain's need for oxygen by reducing oxygen consumption and improving oxygen utilization. Ketones have been shown to protect the brains of lab animals subjected to cerebral hemorrhages or have had their oxygen supply cut off.[59] These animals experience less damage and recover quicker than those without the benefit of ketones. Since many neurological disorders exhibit a decline in brain metabolism, ketones can improve oxygen utilization and protect the brain cells from oxygen starvation. For this reason, intravenous infusion fluids containing ketones are being developed to prevent the cognitive deficits caused by decreased blood flow in the brain during heart bypass surgery.[60]

Our cells use oxygen to convert glucose into energy. When glucose is oxidized into energy, free radicals are formed as byproducts.

Sticking to our automobile analogy, this is similar to when a car burns oxygen and gasoline to produce energy; in the process, toxic exhaust is also produced. In essence, free radicals are the exhaust our cells produce.

Most of the oxygen sent to the brain is used for the conversion of glucose into energy. Since the brain uses an extraordinarily large proportion of the body's oxygen in this process, an exceptionally large amount of free radicals are formed. The brain becomes a hotbed of free-radical activity. In the eyes, this free-radical activity is intensified by exposure to sunlight. Light, especially UV and blue light, are potent free-radical generators. Consequently, the eyes are subjected to an exceptionally high amount of free-radical activity. This is why antioxidants are so important to good eye health and why degenerative eye diseases involve so much free radical-induced damage.

Ketones are like green energy for the body. When cells burn ketones in place of glucose, much less oxygen is used; consequently, free-radical production is greatly reduced and antioxidants are conserved.[61] Ketones produce more energy with far less pollution (free radicals) than glucose. Many of the therapeutic effects of calorie restriction, fasting, and the ketogenic diet are attributed to the substantial reduction in free-radical production.

In addition, when the body is in ketosis, blood glucose is relatively low. This means there is less glucose in the bloodstream that can become glycated and form harmful AGEs. This also reduces the amount of free radicals that may be formed as a result of the AGEs.

One of the most significant effects of ketones on the brain is the activation of neurotrophic factors, BDNF in particular, which play such a critical role in neuron survival and function.[62] When blood glucose levels go down, the liver automatically starts producing ketones as a means to maintain the energy levels required by the brain. Consequently, the ketogenic diet, water-only fasting, intermittent fasting, calorie restriction, and moderate to heavy exercise all reduce blood glucose levels, stimulating the production of ketones. Ketones, in turn, trigger the production and activation of BDNF. Those processes that lower blood glucose the most and raise blood ketones the most, result in the highest levels of BDNF. Mild exercise does not stimulate the production of BDNF, as exercise must be vigorous enough and last long enough to use up stored glycogen and shift the body into a fat-burning state (i.e. reduce blood glucose levels enough to start producing ketones).[63-65] For the same reason, water-only fasting and the ketogenic diet have a greater effect on increasing BDNF than does simple calorie restriction. Type 2 diabetics, who are insulin resistant and have chronic elevated blood sugar levels, have lower than normal BDNF levels.[66] In fact, anyone who is insulin resistant to any degree, including pre-diabetics, will have reduced levels of BDNF. Fortunately, these levels can be increased by increasing blood ketones.

Ketones themselves also appear to protect the brain. Ketones have been shown to increase the survival of acutely damaged rat neocortical neurons in cell cultures exposed to glutamate or hydrogen peroxide for 10 minutes or more. Glutamate toxicity contributes to neuronal degeneration in many central nervous system diseases, including stroke, epilepsy, head trauma, and Alzheimer's.[67]

Sixty percent of the brain consists of lipids (fat and cholesterol). Fats are crucial to proper brain function. Ketones provide the basic lipid building blocks for new brain cells.[68-69] Believe it or not, much of your brain is derived from ketones. The third trimester of pregnancy and the first several months of life are referred to as "the brain growth spurt period." During this time, the brain undergoes its greatest growth and development, and the fetus or infant is in a state of ketosis, having elevated blood ketone levels.[70] Not only do the ketones provide much-needed energy, but they also supply the basic building material for the growing brain. The fully grown adult brain also needs ketones for brain cell synthesis. Brain cells are continually being repaired and replaced, just like other cells in the body. Damaged neurons repair more readily when given an adequate ketone supply.

In summary, ketones play a major role in eye and brain health, and offer many benefits, including:

- Essential for neuron survival
- Provide a high-potency alternative fuel to glucose
- Improve oxygen utilization
- Reduce free-radical formation and conserve antioxidants
- Bypass defects in glucose metabolism or insulin resistance
- Reduce AGE formation
- Activate BDNF to regulate cell growth, repair, and function
- Protect against toxins and stress

- Provide the basic lipid building blocks for repairing damaged brain tissue and generating new brain cells

It's no wonder those who follow a ketogenic diet see so many improvements in overall health! For these reasons, ketones can have a very pronounced effect on brain health and can be used therapeutically to treat brain and eye disorders.

At one time it was believed that the brain could not regenerate. The neurons or brain cells you were born with were all you would ever get; as you grew older, you lost more and more neurons. This idea has long been disproven, for we now know that the brain can and does grow new cells. Likewise, for many years it was also believed that the eyes could not regenerate, but recent discoveries have shown that under the right conditions the retina, optic nerve, and even the photoreceptors can be regenerated.[71-75]

The key to this regeneration is the availability of ketones. Raising blood ketones to therapeutic levels and sustaining these levels for a period of time can set into motion the events that can protect neurons in the brain and eyes from injury and stimulate re-growth. This offers hope, for it means it is possible that vision loss due to age-related eye diseases can potentially be restored, at least to some extent.

9

Coconut Ketones

BETTER BRAIN HEALTH

One morning in December 2012, Vrajlal Parmar got up, washed and dressed himself, and at 10 a.m. boarded the bus to head to a nearby leisure center. In the evening, the 67-year-old former production line worker from London took the bus home.

Nothing about that day would have seemed remarkable if not for the fact that nearly a year earlier, Parmar had been diagnosed with severe late stage Alzheimer's. He had been given a test called the Mini Mental State Exam (MMSE), which doctors use to diagnose and measure the progression of Alzheimer's. A healthy person should be able to answer all 30 questions correctly. A score between 20 and 25 indicates mild dementia, 11 to 19 is moderate dementia, and anything below 10 signifies severe dementia. Parmar was so severely affected that he didn't score anything at all. His condition was so severe that drugs would have no effect.

"Dad was so far gone he couldn't do anything for himself," says his son Kal Parmar, who, together with Vrajlal's wife, Taramati, looks after him at their home in London.

"He couldn't wash himself, dress or go to the toilet without help. He had to be watched all the time—the idea of him catching a bus, even a special bus to a dementia center, was out of the question.

"Often at night he would become hyperactive. We were regularly woken up because Dad was pulling pots and pans off shelves in the kitchen or emptying the cupboards."

146

What has made the difference, according to Kal, is a spoonful of coconut oil twice a day mixed with his food, something the elder Parmar has been taking for about 6 months.

"Before we started him on coconut oil, Dad's speech was gone and he couldn't remember his name or his date of birth. Now you can have a simple conversation with him. We go for walks. He even remembers his national insurance number. We're so happy."

Kal Parmar first heard about using coconut oil in the treatment of Alzheimer's from a video on YouTube—it was about a doctor in Florida who reversed her husband's Alzheimer's using the oil.

Kal says he would probably have dismissed it as just another case of Internet hype if there hadn't been a favorable comment about the oil from Dr. Kieran Clarke, professor of physiological biochemistry at Oxford University and head of the Cardiac Metabolism Research Group.

"That made me think there must be something in it," he says, "so I called her up."

Professor Clarke, an expert on the way the body makes and uses energy, explained to Kal how the MCTs in coconut oil are transformed into ketones in the body. She likens them to a kind of "brain food."

Coconut oil is ketogenic. When it is consumed, a portion of the MCTs in the oil are automatically converted into ketones, regardless of blood sugar levels or what other foods may be in the diet. You can raise blood ketones to therapeutic levels simply by eating coconut oil.[1] In a sense, if you eat enough coconut oil, you can make any diet ketogenic.

Kal began giving his father coconut oil and the results have been incredible.

The doctor from Florida in the YouTube video, Dr. Mary Newport, is a pediatrician who has been using coconut oil with great success to treat her husband, Steve. Alzheimer's doesn't normally surface until sometime after the age of 60. Steve was diagnosed with Alzheimer's at the age of 53. He has what is called early on-set Alzheimer's.

Before the diagnosis, Steve worked as an accountant. Within just a few years, he lost the ability to do simple math, as well as the ability to read or spell simple three-letter words such as "out" or "put." He could no longer type on a keyboard, he had difficultly dressing, and was forgetting family member's names. In addition to his memory problems, he was developing uncontrollable tremors in his hands and face. Walking required slow, labored, mechanical steps.

Dr. Newport gave him all of the standard drugs for Alzheimer's, but they didn't do any good, and the disease continued to progress at a rapid rate. Desperate to find something that might help, she began looking for drugs still in development. Her goal was to enroll Steve in a pilot study intended to test the most promising new drugs. In her search, she came across one particular drug that showed tremendous promise. In preliminary studies with elderly patients suffering from dementia, the medication resulted in measurable improvement in cognitive ability. This was exciting, since no drug had ever shown actual improvement before. None of the drugs on the market can stop the progression of the disease, let alone produce an improvement; at best, they can only slightly slow the progression of this debilitating disease.

Hopeful, Dr. Newport scheduled a screening for Steve so he could participate in the study. At the screening Steve was required to take the Mini Mental State Exam (MMSE). Out of 30 questions, Steve answered only 12 correctly, far below the minimum of 16 required to participate in the study. In fact, his score was so low that it indicated he was approaching the severe stages of Alzheimer's. Steve was considered too far gone, hopeless, and was rejected from the study. Just like that, the Newports were sent home.

Mary had done a lot of research on this drug and in her investigation, she had come across the patent application on the Internet, which detailed the theory and chemistry behind the drug and even included a list of the ingredients. She discovered, that the drug contained only one active ingredient: MCTs derived from coconut oil. Dr. Newport reasoned that if they couldn't participate in the study, they could conduct their own investigation using coconut oil. Mary went to her local health food store and purchased a bottle of virgin coconut oil. She calculated how much coconut oil she would need to give Steve in order to equal the amount of MCTs they were using in the study. It came out to just under two and a half tablespoons.

Two weeks after being rejected from the study, she added this amount of coconut oil into Steve's oatmeal at breakfast. That afternoon they had an appointment with the neurologist. At the appointment

Steve was asked to retake the MMSE test. This time he scored an 18! The improvement was remarkable. The doctor had never seen an Alzheimer's patient improve like that. Alzheimer's is a progressive disease that always gets worse, not better. The Newports knew they had discovered something incredible.

Dr. Newport continued to give Steve coconut oil daily over the next year. In fact, she increased his dosage somewhat to improve his progress. During that time, Steve regained the ability to read, spell, and type. Without assistance, he could log on to the computer and surf the Internet, something he hadn't been able to do for years. His hand and face tremors stopped, and he was able to jog again for the first time in two years. He retook the MMSE test and scored a 20, placing him into the mild range of Alzheimer's. He improved so much that he began volunteering his services at the hospital where his wife was employed, working in the shipping and receiving department.

Steve says that before he started taking coconut oil, he felt as if he was locked in a dark room. He could not think clearly or express himself as he wanted to. When he started taking coconut oil, it was as if someone switched on the light, and he could see and think clearly again. With coconut oil, he says, "I've got my life back!"

Encouraged by her husband's remarkable progress, Dr. Newport conducted an informal study with 60 dementia patients. The purpose of the study was to identify specific improvements in patients with dementia after adding coconut oil/MCTs into their daily diet. The patients' caregivers kept track of and reported the results. The most common improvements occurred in memory, social behavior, speech and conversation, and in daily activities such as reading and doing household chores. Other improvements included reduction in tremors, the ability to walk without assistance, improved strength and balance, increased energy, better sleep, and the reduction in visual disturbance and the ability to see more clearly.[2]

Dr. Newport now travels the country telling Steve's story and encouraging further research in the use of MCTs as a therapeutic aid in treating neurological disorders. Many people with various forms of dementia, Parkinson's, ALS, and other neurodegenerative conditions are incorporating coconut oil into their diets and experiencing remarkable success.

As amazing as these stories are, we don't need to rely on testimonials and reports from caregivers to know that coconut oil can heal the damage caused by various neurological conditions. MCTs have been used successfully to treat—and, in many cases, completely cure—epilepsy since the 1970s. The medical literature is filled with clinical studies demonstrating its use for this purpose.[3-5] MCTs are much more readily converted into ketones than the more common long chain triglycerides. This led to the development of a modified ketogenic diet that relies on MCTs as the primary source of fat. This modified ketogenic diet reduces the total amount of fat needed to induce ketosis and allows a patient to eat a greater amount of carbohydrate and protein, thus broadening dietary choices and improving the palatability and nutritional content of the diet. The modified ketogenic diet has been proven to be just as effective in treating epilepsy as the classic ketogenic diet, a version of which is currently the most common dietary treatment for epilepsy.

In animal studies, dietary supplementation with MCT-based oil has shown to improve the memory of aged dogs.[6] Researchers at Nestle Purina Research in St. Louis, Missouri compared two groups of aged beagles. Cognitive tests at the start of the study showed no difference between the two groups. The diet of one group was supplemented with MCTs for 8 months. Both groups then underwent a battery of cognitive tests to assess learning ability, visuospatial function, and attention. The group that received the MCTs showed significantly better performance as compared to the control group. Because of this and other studies by researchers at Purina and elsewhere, Purina has formulated a commercially available dog food containing coconut oil, geared specifically for older dogs. The company reports that dog owners using the product are noticing improvements in "attention span, trainability, decision making, and overall cognitive function in their pets."

In human studies, MCTs from coconut oil have produced better results in Alzheimer's patients than any other treatment currently in use. In one study, for instance, Alzheimer's patients consumed two beverages, one containing MCTs and one without. Each subject consumed the beverages on different days and took a memory test 90 minutes later. The study found that patients scored significantly better after drinking the beverage containing the MCTs than they did after consuming the beverage without MCTs.[7]

This study is remarkable for three main reasons. First, it proves that MCTs can actually improve cognitive function in Alzheimer's patients. No drug has ever produced a positive effect like this, the very best they can hope do is slow down the progression of the disease slightly, that's all. Second, the effect was seen almost immediately, within 90 minutes the patients were scoring higher on their memory tests. Third, the improvement was achieved after a single dose of MCTs; it did not require 6 months of use or 100 doses in order to see the benefits. No Alzheimer's drug or treatment has ever come close to achieving results like this.

With regular use, coconut oil appears to provide long-term protection for the brain. One of the characteristics in Alzheimer's is the formation of amyloid plaque deposits in brain tissue. We all develop some amyloid plaque deposits in our brains as we age. Those with Alzheimer's, however, accumulate five to ten times more than normal. This plaque begins to form in areas important for learning and memory and eventually spreads to other regions in the brain. It is believed to be an important contributor to the mental degeneration seen in Alzheimer's patients. Coconut oil has been shown to prevent the formation of amyloid plaque deposits in brain tissue. In tissue cultures when amyloid plaque is combined with healthy brain tissue, the plaque spreads, affecting the entire culture. Researchers have shown that when coconut oil is added to these cultures it stops the growth of the plaque dead cold.[8] This suggests that coconut oil not only helps to prevent the plaque that overruns the Alzheimer's brain, but it may also be able to reduce the amount that develops during normal aging, thus helping to preserve normal brain function as we grow older.

MCTs have shown to attenuate the symptoms of ALS, a neurodegenerative motor neuron disease. Researchers at Mount Sinai School of Medicine in New York City tested MCTs on mice genetically bred to develop ALS. Feeding the mice MCTs protected them against the motor neuron loss that accompanies the clinical symptoms of ALS and increased their survival time.[9]

ALS patients who include coconut oil as part of their treatment are also seeing benefits. Butch Matchlin was officially diagnosed with

ALS in September of 2008. He started a journal to keep track of his symptoms and monitor the progress of the disease. His mother died of ALS in 1986, after suffering for 8 years with the loss of all muscle functions, including her ability speak. For over a year, she had to rely on a respirator to breathe, and during the last two to three months of her life, nearly all the muscles of her body were immobile. Sadly, her only method of communicating was by blinking and moving her eyes. Butch's original motivation for keeping the journal was to compare his symptoms to his mother's, so he would be prepared for each step in the process.

In late 2009 Butch started taking 3 tablespoons of coconut oil daily. This amount gradually increased over the next couple of years. To the disbelief of his doctors, during that time the progression of his disease suddenly stopped and many of his symptoms began to improve. His detailed journal documents his condition before starting coconut oil and afterward. Two and a half years after he began using coconut oil he notes that his muscle strength has improved. He noticed increased size and strength in his leg muscles, improved mobility in his toes and feet, and the ability to perform many tasks with greater ease than he had previously, such as rolling over in bed and putting on his shoes. He had no more muscle cramps, spasms, or insomnia. He still has difficulty moving about, but his condition is greatly improved from what it was, results that are unheard of in cases of ALS, a disease that is always progressive and ultimately fatal. Although coconut oil has not cured Butch, it has made his life a whole lot easier.

MCTs have an overall healing effect on the brain. Hospital patients who cannot eat, for one reason or another, are often given nutritional formulas administered intravenously (IV). When patients who have suffered severe head trauma are given nutritional IV emulsions containing MCTs, recovery is significantly enhanced.[10-11]

Since the eyes are extensions of the brain, diseases of the brain can have an effect on vision. People who suffer from neurological disorders often experience visual problems. In Alzheimer's patients, for example, visual problems are often among the earliest complaints.[12] The reduction in energy metabolism (i.e., insulin resistance) seen in most neurodegenerative conditions has an effect on the retina and optic nerve. In Alzheimer's patients there is a marked narrowing of the retinal blood vessels and a reduction in blood flow, resulting in degeneration of the retina and optic nerve.[13] A decrease in retina and macular volume correlates with the increasing severity of the disease,[14] though the degeneration in vision varies from patient to patient.

Because coconut oil increases blood levels of ketones, much like the ketogenic diet, consuming the oil can bring about much of the same benefits on brain and nerve health. People who add coconut oil into their daily diets report improvements in a number of neurological conditions including epilepsy, Alzheimer's, ALS, Parkinson's, MS, depression, autism, glaucoma, and retinopathy.

Because coconut oil is ketogenic, just adding the oil into your regular diet can bring about definite improvements in brain and overall health. However, in order to duplicate the same level of benefit associated with a ketogenic diet, coconut oil should be consumed with a low-carb diet. Consuming too many carbs will raise blood glucose levels, promote insulin resistance, and increase AGE formation and free-radical activity, all of which are detrimental to healthy brain and eye function.

ADDING COCONUT OIL INTO YOUR LIFE

You have learned about the many benefits of coconut oil, and it should be obvious that this extraordinary brain food can play a vital role in the fight against neurodegenerative disorders. Therefore, understanding how to incorporate it into your daily life is important. The simplest way to do this is to prepare your meals with it. Coconut oil is very heat stable, so it is excellent for use in the kitchen, for any baking or frying you do. In recipes that call for margarine, butter, shortening, or vegetable oil, use coconut oil instead. Use the same amount or more to make sure you get the recommended amount in your diet.

Not all foods are prepared using oil, but you can still incorporate the oil into the diet. Coconut oil can be added to all foods, even if they do not call for oil. For example, add a spoonful of coconut oil to hot beverages, hot cereals, soups, sauces, and casseroles, or use it as a topping on cooked vegetables.

Although I recommend that you consume coconut oil with food, you don't have to prepare your food with it or add it to the food. If you prefer, you can take it by the spoonful, like a dietary supplement.

Many people prefer to get their daily dose of coconut oil this way. If you use a good quality coconut oil, it will taste good. On the other hand, putting a whole spoonful of oil in the mouth may take some getting used to.

There are two primary types of coconut oil you will find sold in stores. One is called virgin coconut oil and the other refined, bleached, deodorized (RBD) coconut oil. Virgin coconut oil is made from fresh coconuts, with very minimal processing. This oil basically comes straight from the coconut. Since it has gone through little processing, it retains a delicate coconut taste and aroma, and it is delicious.

RBD coconut oil is made from copra (air-dried coconut) and has gone through more extensive processing. During the processing all the flavor and aroma has been removed. For those who do not like the taste of coconut, RBD oil is a good option. RBD oil is processed using mechanical means and high temperatures, chemicals are not generally used. When you go to the store, you can tell the difference between virgin and RBD coconut oils by the label. All virgin coconut oils will state that they are "virgin." RBD oils will not have this statement. They also do not say "RBD." Sometimes they will be advertised as "Expeller Pressed," which means the initial pressing of the oil from the coconut meat was done mechanically, without the use of heat. However, heat is usually used at some later stage in the refining process.

Many people prefer virgin coconut oil because it has undergone less processing and retains more of the nutrients and the flavor nature put into it. This is why it maintains its coconut flavor. Because more care is taken to produce virgin coconut oil, it is more expensive than RBD oil.

Most brands of RBD oil are generally tasteless and odorless and differ little from each other. The quality of the different brands of virgin coconut oil, however, can vary greatly. There are many different processing methods used to produce virgin coconut oil. Some are better than others. The care taken also affects the quality. Some companies produce excellent coconut oil that tastes so good you can easily eat it off a spoon. Other brands have a strong flavor and may be nearly unpalatable. You generally cannot tell the difference just by looking at the jar. You have to taste it. If the oil has a mild coconut flavor and smell, and tastes good to you, then that is a brand you should use. If the flavor is overpowering or smells smoky, you might want to try another brand.

Coconut oil is available at all health food stores and many grocery stores, as well as on the Internet. There are many different brands to choose from. Generally the more expensive brands are the best quality, but not always. The cheaper brands of virgin coconut oil are almost always of inferior quality. All brands, however, have basically the same culinary and therapeutic effects and are useful.

If you purchase coconut oil from the store, it may have the appearance of shortening, firm and white in color. When you take it home and put it on your kitchen shelf, it may transform into a colorless liquid after a few days. If this occurs, don't be alarmed, for it is entirely natural. One of the distinctive characteristics of coconut oil is its high melting point. At temperatures of 76 degrees F (24 degrees C) and above the oil is liquid, like any other vegetable oil. At lower temperatures, it solidifies. It is much like butter; if you store it in the refrigerator, it will solidify, but if you leave it on the counter on a hot day, it will melt into a puddle. It will be safe no matter how you choose to store it, and you can use it in either form.

Coconut oil is very stable, so it does not need to be refrigerated. You can store it on a cupboard shelf. Shelf life for a good-quality coconut oil is 1 to 3 years. Hopefully, you will use it long before then.

MCT OIL

Most of the health benefits associated with coconut oil come from its medium chain triglycerides. If MCTs are good, it can be reasoned that a source that contains more than coconut oil may be even better. Coconut oil is the richest "natural" source of MCTs, but there is another source that contains more: MCT oil. Coconut oil consists of 63 percent MCTs, while MCT oil is 100 percent. MCT oil, which is sometimes referred to as "fractionated coconut oil," is produced from coconut oil. The 10 fatty acids that make up coconut oil are separated out, and two of the medium chain fatty acids (caprylic and capric acids) are recombined to form MCT oil.

The advantage of MCT oil is that it provides more MCTs per volume than coconut oil. It is tasteless and, since it is liquid at room temperature, it can easily be used as a salad dressing or mixed into cold drinks. The disadvantage of MCT oil is that it can only be used in low-temperature cooking because it burns easily. It is more likely to cause nausea and diarrhea than coconut oil, and it can only be used in a limited amount without causing these undesirable side effects.

MCT oil contains no lauric acid, the most important of the medium chain fatty acids. In contrast, nearly 50 percent of coconut oil consists of lauric acid. Lauric acid possesses the most potent antimicrobial power. When combined with the other fatty acids in the oil, the naturally strong antimicrobial potential of lauric acid is only enhanced. Consequently, coconut oil has a far greater germ-fighting ability than MCT oil.

The MCFAs in MCT oil are quickly converted into ketones. Blood ketone levels peak 1½ hours after consumption and are gone after 3 hours. The conversion of lauric acid into ketones is slower. Ketone levels peak at 3 hours after consumption of coconut oil, but remain in the blood for about 8 hours. MCT oil may give a quicker and higher peak in ketosis, but fizzles out much sooner. This is important to consider, because neurons in the brain and eyes need a continual supply of ketones throughout the day and night for best therapeutic effect.

MCT oil would need to be administered every 2 hours or so, day and night, to maintain blood ketone levels. During sleep, brain function remains fully active and needs energy just as much as when you are fully awake. You would need to be awakened constantly throughout the night to take doses of MCT oil. This amount of MCT oil is unrealistic because of the undesirable digestive disturbances it would cause.

Coconut oil, on the other hand, only needs to be taken three or four times a day and can last throughout the night. Some people who had been using coconut oil to treat Alzheimer's but switched to using only MCT oil reported a decline in progress. The conclusion is that MCT oil can be added to a treatment program but should not completely replace coconut oil. Although MCT oil may produce a quicker rise in ketosis, it really isn't necessary. Coconut oil lasts longer, has fewer side effects, and is more effective in treating infections.

Another type of oil you may find at the market is "liquid" or "winterized" coconut oil. This oil has the longer chain fatty acids removed. It is very similar to MCT oil in its fatty acid profile, but with a slightly greater mix of different fatty acids. It, too, has a lower melting point than ordinary coconut oil and can be used on cold foods without hardening, and like MCT oil, it is not the best for cooking.

10

Coconut Therapy

AGE-RELATED EYE DISORDERS

Cataracts, glaucoma, macular degeneration, diabetic retinopathy, and other age-related eye disorders share many common characteristics. Among these are high oxidative stress and free-radical damage, low levels of protective antioxidant nutrients and enzymes, high polyunsaturated fatty acid levels in tissues, chronically high blood sugar levels or insulin resistance, chronic inflammation, and tissue degeneration.

Age-related eye diseases are not actually caused by aging as we think of it; rather, they are the result of years of exposure to destructive conditions that prematurely age and damage the eye. People can live long, healthy lives without experiencing these so-called age-related diseases. The eyes of healthy seniors who age normally are very different from the eyes of people of any age who suffer from cataracts, macular degeneration, and other degenerative eye diseases.

Age-related eye diseases are primarily the result of diet and lifestyle choices. Consequently, they can be avoided, stopped, and even reversed to some degree by making the appropriate changes now, whatever stage of life you are in. The changes include things you should avoid that promote aging and vision loss and things you should be doing to preserve and restore your vision.

Nutritious Diet

If your eyes are to be healthy and provide you with a lifetime of good service, you must provide them with the nutrients they need to function properly. This means you must eat nutrient-dense foods and avoid filling up on poor-quality foods such as sweets and refined carbohydrates (bread, donuts, chips, crackers, cookies) and other junk foods. Nutrient-dense foods are whole foods like fresh vegetables, fruits, nuts, meats, eggs, and dairy. These healthier choices will provide you with the essential vitamins, minerals, and antioxidants your eyes need to maintain good health.

It is interesting that the foods that provide the fewest nutrients are generally the richest in simple carbohydrates. They quickly raise blood sugar levels and promote insulin resistance. These and other highly processed foods are also more likely to be contaminated with harmful food additives such as aspartame and MSG.

One of the major contributors to all forms of degenerative eye disease is excessive oxidative stress. A diet low in antioxidant nutrients cannot provide the protection the eyes demand. The eyes are exposed to a much higher level of oxidation than other parts of the body, and a poor diet has more of an adverse effect on the eyes than it will on other tissues that do not require as many antioxidants.

Fresh vegetables are often recommended as excellent sources of the nutrients vital to good eye health. However, as you read in Chapter 7, if you don't consume vegetables along with a good source of fat, you won't absorb their nutrients, especially the fat-soluble ones such as beta-carotene, lutein, and zeaxanthin. While any fat will improve nutrient absorption, coconut oil has been shown to be the most effective. Just adding coconut oil to a meal can double, triple, or quadruple the nutrient value of vegetables, providing the eyes with that much more protection.

Studies consistently show that diets rich in essential vitamins and minerals and protective antioxidants delay the development and progression of degenerative eye diseases. However, they have not shown to be effective in stopping or reversing these diseases. To achieve that, you must control blood sugar and stimulate the repair process with ketones. Multivitamin supplements, even those with lutein and zeaxanthin, won't do a bit of good if your diet is loaded with sugar and refined carbs.

Control Blood Sugar

High-sugar diets and those high in refined carbohydrates promote vision degeneration. High carb consumption leads to chronic high blood glucose levels, which in turn, leads to insulin resistance.

Insulin resistance develops in people who eat high-carb diets consisting principally of sweets and refined grains. After consumption, the carbs are converted into glucose and sent into the bloodstream. If a large amount of carbs are eaten throughout the day, blood glucose levels remain elevated most of the time. Constant exposure to high blood glucose levels over a period of many years desensitizes the cells to the action of insulin, resulting in insulin resistance.

Insulin resistance slows the rate at which glucose can enter the cells. Consequently, blood glucose levels rise to abnormally high levels and remain elevated for an extended period of time. One of the problems with this is that glucose tends to glycate, or stick to proteins and fats in the bloodstream, creating harmful AGEs, which stimulate the production of destructive free radicals. One of the characteristics of diabetes, and a problem with those who suffer from age-related eye disease, is runaway free-radical degeneration throughout the body, including the eyes.

Another problem, one more serious, is the inability of the cells to properly absorb glucose, which is the fuel required for cells to function properly. Without it, they die. Our cells need a continual supply of glucose to maintain their health. When glucose delivery is slowed by insulin resistance, the function of the cells slows too. If the cells do not get enough glucose, they begin to starve, degenerate, and die. This process of cell death is most notable in the blood vessels and capillaries. As the cells in the circulatory system begin to degenerate, they become leaky, and blood and oxygen delivery to peripheral tissues declines. Starved of blood and oxygen, these tissues also begin to die, and this leads to many of the complications associated with diabetes, such as peripheral neuropathy (numbness in the feet and legs), retinopathy (blindness), and nephropathy (kidney failure). Poor circulation and blood clots are often associated with diabetes, putting diabetics at very high risk for heart attacks and strokes.

When insulin resistance is severe, it causes diabetes. Diabetes is diagnosed when fasting blood sugar—the blood glucose levels after an 8 hour fast—reaches 126 mg/dl (7 mmol/l) or more. In a healthy individual, fasting blood sugar levels are generally no greater than 90 mg/dl (5.0 mmol/l); any higher indicates some level of insulin resistance and all the problems associated with it. The higher the blood sugar level, the greater the damage. Chronic fasting blood sugar levels over 90 mg/dl increase your risk of degenerative eye disease, not only because of the deterioration of tiny blood vessels and capillaries in your eyes, but also because it greatly increases your exposure to damaging free radicals, AGEs, and inflammation.

Diabetics and even pre-diabetics are at very high risk of developing dementia because insulin resistance affects brain health and function. As mentioned previously, Alzheimer's disease is now considered a form of diabetes. Parkinson's disease is also associated with insulin resistance. Essentially, all degenerative brain diseases involve some level of insulin resistance, and this appears to be true for age-related eye diseases as well.[1-4] Those people who eat higher amounts of carbohydrate are at a significantly greater risk of developing macular degeneration, cataracts, retinopathy, and other age-related eye disorders. As an example, a study at Tufts University in Boston showed that eating foods with an above-average glycemic index was associated with a 49 percent increase in advanced macular degeneration.[5] The glycemic index measures how quickly certain foods raise blood sugar levels. Those that raise blood sugar levels the most, like bread and sugar, are the most detrimental. Dr. Allen Taylor, the lead researcher in that study, reports that the results indicated that at least one in five cases of advanced AMD (the only eye disease evaluated in the study) could likely have been prevented entirely by consuming fewer carbs. Similarly, studies show that when blood sugar is not well controlled it leads to cataracts, but when blood sugar is kept under control, cataracts can be prevented.[6]

Therefore, one of the first steps in preventing and stopping age-related eye disease is to take control of your fasting blood sugar levels with a goal of staying consistently below 91 mg/dl or as close to it as you possibly can. This is doable even if you are diabetic. You can accomplish this by eating a low-carb or ketogenic diet, as discussed in detail in the following chapter.

Another measurement used to test for insulin resistance is the glycated hemoglobin or A1C test. This test measures how much hemoglobin has been glycated—a measure of AGEs in the blood. It reveals your average blood sugar level over the past three months. The higher your blood sugar levels, the more glycated hemoglobin you will have. An A1C level of 6.5 percent or higher, measured in two separate tests, indicates the presence of diabetes. An A1C between 5.7 and 6.4 percent indicates pre-diabetes. Below 5.7 is considered normal or typical, but this doesn't necessarily mean healthy. A reading of 5.0 or lower is a better goal to shoot for.

Coconut Oil and Insulin Resistance

Coconut oil works wonders for alleviating symptoms associated with diabetes and insulin resistance. Studies show that MCTs improve insulin secretion and insulin sensitivity.[7] When added to meals, dietary fat—and coconut oil in particular—slows the absorption of sugar into the bloodstream, thus moderating blood sugar levels. Eaten with meals, coconut oil can be very effective in keeping blood sugar under control. Even when taken after or between meals, it can help lower elevated blood sugar.

This effect reduces the need for insulin injections. Some diabetics have discovered that taking coconut oil even eliminates their need for additional insulin. "Virgin coconut oil has a substantial effect on blood sugar levels," says Ed. "My wife and daughter (both have type 2 diabetes) measure their blood sugar levels at least three times a day. When they eat the wrong foods and their blood sugar levels get to 80 to 100 points above normal, they don't take extra medication, they take 2 to 3 tablespoons of coconut oil directly from the bottle. Within a half hour their blood sugar levels will come back to normal."

"I was diagnosed as type 2 diabetic in July of 2001 and immediately put on the Amaryl RX," says Sharon. "I have been looking for a way to reverse this condition since diagnosed. I have found a world of info out there on various supplements and diet. BUT not from my doctor, who just said, 'Welcome to the club,' and told me to take my meds. (I was crying and he seemed happy!)... Bottom line is this. I have been able to slowly remove myself from the RX and now control my blood sugar by diet, supplements, and with coconut oil! Cool, huh? I do still check my blood sugar levels once or twice daily and they are as good, and usually better, than when I was on the Amaryl RX!"

Coconut oil does more than just balance blood sugar, it can actually reverse damage caused by insulin resistance. Diabetic neuropathy is a condition in which nerves are damaged due to the degeneration of tiny blood vessels and capillaries, particularly in peripheral tissues. The effects are felt as pain or numbness in the feet and legs. Other symptoms include digestive problems, muscle weakness and cramps, loss of bladder control, dizziness, speech impairment, and degeneration of vision. Approximately 50 percent of diabetics will eventually develop nerve damage.

Poor circulation in the extremities is a common cause of diabetic foot ulcers that can lead to gangrene and amputation. Because of poor circulation, relatively minor cuts or injuries on the feet or legs of a diabetic can persist for months and become gangrenous. If the limb is numb, the injury and accompanying infection and decay can be painless.

Poor circulation results from degeneration of blood vessels and capillaries caused by the inability of the cells to properly absorb glucose. Insulin resistance impedes glucose transport into the cells, causing them to slowly degenerate and die. Coconut oil can help revive diseased and dying tissues by boosting blood levels of ketones. Ketones do not require insulin to enter the cells, so they are not affected by insulin resistance. When ketones are available, they pass easily into the cells of blood vessels and capillaries, keeping them alive and promote healing and renewed growth, thus improving circulation, restoring life to nerves, and reversing the complications often associated with diabetes. The ketogenic diet, which increases blood ketones, has proven to actually reverse diabetic nephropathy (kidney disease). Studies also prove that while lowering blood sugar does stop the progression of nephropathy, it alone cannot reverse it. Raising blood ketones is necessary for the reversal. [8]

Many diabetics have experienced the reawaking of nearly dead limbs when they added coconut oil into their diets. "I did have a minor scrape on my lower right leg that has been trying to heal for a couple of months," says Edward K. "My wife called it an ugly wound. Six years ago my feet started to get numb, starting with the large toe and, over the years, the feet would become more and more numb. I began taking around 3 to 4 tablespoons per day of coconut oil. Within 10 days the injury on my leg healed up totally. I am so happy because now I feel the feeling coming back. The numbness is leaving. I have more feeling now."

Edward was at serious risk of having his wound become infected and perhaps eventually undergoing surgery or amputation. In just 10 days coconut oil healed the blood vessels in his feet and legs, improving his circulation, allowing the cut to completely heal, and brought life back into legs and feet. Edward's story isn't unusual; many diabetics experience the same response when they start taking coconut oil regularly.

The eyes can also benefit. "My retinopathy has been completely gone for three years now," says Kim. "I've added more fat into my diet, in the way of coconut oil and other healthy fats, which have helped greatly in controlling my blood sugar [levels]. Even though they weren't too bad before, they are even better now."

Coconut oil improves circulation and reverses blood vessel and nerve damage in the extremities. It can do the same in the brain and eyes. Every diabetic and anyone with any degree of insulin resistance could benefit from using coconut oil on a regular basis.

Ketone Power

Blood sugar control is vital if you want to prevent or stop the progression of degenerative eye disease, but that alone will not repair the damage or reverse the condition. Oxidative stress and inflammation contribute to the development of degenerative eye disease and prevent healing, even after good glycemic control is reinstated. Here is where ketones come into play. Ketones reduce oxidative stress and inflammation and activate BDNF that stimulate healing, repair, and growth of new neurons in the brain and eyes. Ketones have proven useful in healing a variety of brain disorders ranging from epilepsy to Alzheimer's.

Ketones are actually vital to healthy brain and eye function. Glucose is the main source of fuel for the brain, primarily because blood glucose levels rise whenever we eat a meal or snack. However, if we don't eat for several hours, blood glucose levels can drop low enough that the liver begins to convert stored fat into ketones. During these times the brain relies heavily on ketones to meet its energy needs. Ketones ease free-radical stress, pump up BDNF, and initiate much of the maintenance, healing, and repair needed to keep the brain and eyes in good working order.

It is much like buying a new car. When you take that car off the parking lot it has the potential to give you many years of reliable service. However, in order to get the most from that car you need to take care of it, rotate the tires, change the air and fuel filters, and change the oil regularly. If you do these things, your car will easily give you over 100,000 miles of reliable service. However, if you neglect to perform these routine maintenance procedures, you will be lucky to get 20,000 miles before the engine seizes up and the car breaks down and dies.

Our brains and eyes are similar. At birth, they have the potential to provide us with over 100 years of reliable service—if we take care of them. Ketones are like the mechanics who come in and change the oil and rotate the tires. They keep our brains in good working order throughout the course of our lifetime. For this to happen, though, blood ketone levels must be elevated periodically.

The types of foods we eat, along with meal frequency strongly affect how often and how many ketones we produce and the effect they have on brain and eye health. Some people produce little or none, thus losing out on their potential therapeutic effect.

What types of foods do you eat every day? Does the following list sound familiar? For breakfast: hot or cold cereal, muffins, toast, pancakes, waffles, fruit, or juice. For lunch: a sandwich, burrito, hamburger, fries, onion rings, or chips. For a snack: a granola bar, donut, coffee with sugar. For dinner: pizza, pasta, potatoes, and bread, finished with a dessert of cake, pie, or ice cream. All of these foods are high in carbohydrates, which are easily transformed into glucose in the body. If you eat like this, your blood sugar levels will be elevated essentially all day long, and your body will never have an opportunity to produce any significant amount of ketones.

If you are already insulin resistant, that means your blood sugar remains elevated even when you are not eating. So even after you wake up in the morning and have not eaten for 12 hours, your blood sugar levels will be elevated. This means your body's ketone-making machine is never activated. If you eat like this every day, day after day, year after year, your brain and eyes will age at an accelerated rate, resulting in some level of neurodegenerative disease. This is why BDNF are significantly lower in diabetics as compared to non-diabetics.[9]

The best medicine for the prevention and treatment of any age-related eye disease is to allow your body to increase its ketone levels on a regular basis. The higher and the longer you can maintain elevated ketone levels, the better. You can accomplish this by fasting, eating a ketogenic diet, or by adding an adequate amount of coconut oil into your daily diet.

Brain-Derived Neurotrophic Factors

For many years it was believed that abnormally high intraocular pressure was the primary cause of glaucoma. However, some researchers are now reassessing this belief. While excessive intraocular pressure is involved, it may not be the actual cause of retinal ganglion cell and optic nerve degeneration; in fact, it may only be a symptom rather than the initiating factor.

The treatments for glaucoma have focused solely on lowering the intraocular pressure. This approach, unfortunately, often turns out to be unsuccessful; thus suggesting the involvement of other factors or mechanisms in the initiation and or progression of the disease.[10] Even when surgery or medication successfully lowers intraocular pressure, vision loss continues in some glaucoma patients.

Many researchers now view glaucoma as a neurologic disorder that causes nerve cells in the brain to degenerate and die, similar to what occurs in Parkinson's or Alzheimer's.[11] Chronic inflammation, characteristic of all neurodegenerative disorders, is now becoming recognized as an important factor in glaucoma. In Parkinson's disease the area of the brain called the substantia nigra, which controls movement, is affected most. In Alzheimer's, it affects the hippocampus and frontal lobes, areas that involve memory. In glaucoma, it is the eyes.

Damage to, and death of cells in the retina, mimics the degeneration in brain cells. In fact, the same type of plaque that forms in an Alzheimer's brain also forms in the retina. Studies show that Alzheimer's patients have an increased risk of developing glaucoma. A German study of institutionalized Alzheimer's patients showed a 24.5 percent increased prevalence of glaucoma compared to only 6.5 percent of age-matched patients without the disease.[12] A Japanese study showed similar results: Alzheimer's patients had an increased prevalence of glaucoma of 23.8 percent compared to control patients with 9.9 percent.[13] Not only are Alzheimer's patients more likely to develop glaucoma, but glaucoma patients are also at increased risk of developing Alzheimer's. A study of 812 glaucoma subjects, 72 years of age and older, found that they were four times more likely to develop dementia.[14]

While intraocular pressure is an important diagnostic tool and reducing abnormal pressure is still the standard form of treatment, researchers are looking at new approaches. One of these is to take advantage of the body's own healing mechanisms—neurotrophic factors. BDNF are known to protect and revitalize retinal ganglion cells, even causing new cells to grow and repair a damaged optic nerve. Initial studies using rats with glaucoma have shown that when BDNF were injected into the vitreous humor of their eyes, retinal cell degeneration and loss abruptly declined.[15] However, this effect was only temporary. Multiple injections were necessary for significant beneficial effect, reducing the clinical usefulness of this approach. A continuous supply of BDNF is necessary for a beneficial outcome. While injecting BDNF may not be practical, raising and sustaining blood levels of BDNF naturally with a ketogenic or coconut oil-based diet, is very doable and has given amazing results for those with Alzheimer's and other neurodegenerative diseases.

Mary Newport, MD has advocated the use of coconut oil and MCTs as a treatment for neurodegenerative disease ever since she used it to reverse her husband's Alzheimer's. Although her focus is on Alzheimer's, she has noted that a variety of neurodegenerative diseases respond well to the use of coconut oil, including eye disorders, such as glaucoma. She says, "The eyes are an extension of the brain, and neurons are involved in diseases like glaucoma and macular degeneration. This lady who has glaucoma, said that she took MCT oil, and she happened to be sitting at her computer, and she thought that the screen was shades of gray. She thought that was the normal screen. The screen became pink. She started seeing color on the screen, and it was news to her that it was even in color. She thought, 'Well, that's rather odd.' So she repeated this experiment several days in a row, and every time she'd take the MCT oil, about a half hour to 45 minutes later her screen would come in color. I thought that was pretty interesting. She's kept in touch with me too, and about a year and half now, her glaucoma's been stable. She hasn't gotten worse."

While researching AMD, Marlene G. discovered coconut oil. "At the age of 51, I was diagnosed with macular degeneration," says Marlene. "I asked my ophthalmologist if there was anything I can do to reverse it and he flatly said 'No!'" Shocked by his answer, Marlene began a search that led her to coconut oil. "I started taking 2 tablespoons of coconut oil with my breakfast each morning and began using it for cooking. The following year, on my return to the same doctor he discovered I no longer had macular degeneration!" The doctor was dumbfounded, he had no explanation.

Coconut oil may help even when it is used topically as an eyedrop solution. Robert P. reports, "Coconut oil in my wife's eyes reversed her tunnel vision due to glaucoma. It took 30 years to develop tunnel vision and a couple of weeks to heal the nerve damage. Of course she is really happy I don't have to lead her around anymore." A combination of consuming the oil and using it in the eyes, along with a low-carb diet, may be the best natural approach for treating glaucoma and other age-related eye diseases.

Five Steps to Beat Age-Related Eye Disorders
The most important concepts you should know and understand, to avoid or treat age-related degenerative eye diseases, can be boiled down to just five basic steps, each of which is summarized below.

(1) Keep blood sugar levels under control. All degenerative eye disorders are adversely affected by high blood sugar levels. High blood sugar contributes to premature aging of the eyes, either as the underlying cause or as a major contributing factor. Strive to bring your fasting blood sugar levels below 101 mg/dl (5.6 mmol/l) and ideally below 91 mg/dl (5.1 mmol/l). Blood sugar is best controlled by eating a low-carb or ketogenic diet, as explained in the following chapter.

(2) Eat good sources of essential vitamins and antioxidants. Your diet should include ample dark green, red, yellow, and orange vegetables and fruits, along with fresh eggs, meat, and dairy. Avoid highly processed, packaged foods and food additives such as aspartame, MSG, hydrogenated vegetable oils, and polyunsaturated vegetable oils.

168

(3) Raise blood ketone levels. There are a number of ways you can increase blood ketones: periodic water-only fasting, intermittent fasting, regular moderate to heavy aerobic exercise, eating a ketogenic diet, or consuming coconut oil. You can do these separately or combine them for greater effect; for example, eating a ketogenic diet with coconut oil and regular exercise.

(4) Eat good fats. These include coconut, palm, MCT, olive, and macadamia nut oils, as well as butter, cream, and animal fats. Of these, coconut and MCT oils are the only ones that can raise blood ketone levels. Coconut and palm oil are among the best for cooking. Avoid vegetable oils that have a high polyunsaturated fat content such as corn, soybean, safflower, sunflower, peanut, walnut, and canola oils and also all hydrogenated or partially hydrogenated oils.

(5) Avoid drugs. Many prescription and over-the-counter drugs adversely affect eye heath, so you should, to the best of your ability, stop all unnecessary medications. Eating a coconut oil-based, low-carb or ketogenic diet will eliminate the need for most drugs. Such a diet will also balance blood sugar, improve cholesterol and triglyceride levels, normalize high blood pressure, reduce inflammation (C-reactive protein), improve sleep, reduce the risk of heart disease, and help lose excess weight—conditions the vast majority of drugs are designed to treat. Simply eating the right way can eliminate the need for these drugs.

NEURODEGENERATIVE DISEASE

Neurodegenerative diseases like Alzheimer's, Parkinson's, MS, and stroke can adversely affect vision. Although one specific area of the central nervous system may be affected more than others, chronic inflammation and oxidative stress associated with these conditions can affect the entire brain.

The five basic steps to beat age-related eye disorders described above, are also applicable for neurodegenerative disease. Coconut oil, ketones, and a low-carb diet have proven very successful in reversing the symptoms associated with neurodegeneration. If you would like to learn more about the use of coconut oil and diet to beat these diseases, I recommend reading my book *Stop Alzheimer's Now!: How to Prevent and Reverse Dementia, Parkinson's, ALS, Multiple Sclerosis, and Other Neurodegenerative Disorders*.

COCONUT WATER AND CATARACTS

When you walk through the produce aisle in the grocery store, you are sure to run across a stack of brown, hairy coconuts. If you pick one up, shake it, and listen closely, you will hear a swishing sound. Inside the hollow chamber of the coconut is a liquid called coconut water. Some people refer to this as "coconut milk," but this is really a misnomer, since coconut milk is an entirely different product made by crushing coconut meat and extracting the juice. Coconut milk is a thick, white, creamy liquid that looks like dairy milk, while coconut water is a mostly clear liquid that looks much like ordinary water.

In recent years, coconut water has become very popular and is often used as a natural rehydration beverage by athletes and fitness enthusiasts. Coconut water is superior to commercial sports drinks for several reasons. It contains no added sugar, preservatives, emulsifiers, or other chemicals and contains a full spectrum of electrolytes (mineral ions) similar to those present in human blood plasma. It also contains a variety of vitamins, antioxidants, and phytonutrients.

Included with these phytonutrients are plant hormones known as cytokinins, which regulate plant growth and differentiation. Cytokinins have gained keen interest among researchers due to their anti-aging effects in both plants and animals, including humans.

One of the ways cytokinins retard the effects of aging is by blocking one of the major factors involved in the aging process—free radicals. Cytokinins are potent antioxidants. While the antioxidant properties of cytokinins are important and helpful, they are not the primary means by which aging is affected. One of the primary functions of cytokinins is to regulate cell division and influence the rate at which plants age. Depending on the amount of cytokinins present, the aging process in plants can either be accelerated or retarded. One active site of cytokinin production is in the roots. From there, the hormone is carried, via the sap, throughout the plant. Portions of plants that are deprived of a continuous supply of cytokinins age faster than normal. Conversely, if additional cytokinins are added to a plant, normal aging is retarded.

Preserving living tissue for culture studies or transplantation is important to researchers and physicians. In order to ensure tissue quality at a later time, they are stored in special solutions that keep them alive and viable. Coconut water has been shown to be effective in prolonging the life of human and animal tissues.[16] In fact, it is even more effective than Braun-Collins solution and other common storage media that have been formulated specifically for this purpose.[17-18]

As they age, normal human cells go through a progressive, irreversible accumulation of changes, until they reach the stage of death. Young cells are plump, round, and smooth. As they age, they become irregular in shape, flatten out, enlarge, and fill up with debris; cell division slows and eventually stops, which is ultimately followed by death. When cytokinins are added to the culture medium, cells don't act their age. The normal sequence of aging slows down considerably. Cells do not undergo the severe degenerative changes that ordinarily occur.[19-20] Although the total lifespan of human cells is not affected much, the cells remain significantly more youthful and functional throughout their lifetime. For example, treated cells, after they have reached the final stage of their lifespan and no longer divide, look and function like untreated cells half their age. Treated cells never undergo the severe degenerative changes experienced by untreated cells. In all respects, their youth is extended into old age.

Investigators theorize that because of the antioxidant and anti-aging properties of cytokinins, they may have potential in the prevention and treatment of medical conditions such as cancer, heart disease, cataracts, macular degeneration, and Alzheimer's disease. For this reason, the use of coconut water may prove beneficial in preventing some of these conditions. Studies show that in both tissue cultures and living lab animals, coconut water prevents the neurotoxic effects of amyloid plaque formation associated with Alzheimer's disease.[21-22]

Kinetin is the most thoroughly studied cytokinin with anti-aging properties. Because of kinetin's anti-aging effects on plant, animal, and human cells, it has been tested as a topical ointment for the possible treatment for age spots, wrinkles, and sagging, dry, or rough skin. One of the factors that cause wrinkles and sagging skin is the aging and breakdown of connective tissues in the skin. Connective tissues give the skin strength and elasticity. When kinetin is applied to the skin, it stimulates cell division of connective tissue, and this replaces older, damaged tissue with functionally younger tissue.[23] As a result, wrinkled and sagging skin tend to flatten and firm up. Dry, aging skin is replaced with smoother, softer skin.

Topical solutions containing kinetin have also been shown to reduce or normalize abnormal pigmentation such as age spots.[24] In studies on human subjects lasting up to 100 days, no adverse effects have been reported; therefore, kinetin is considered safe to use for long-term application. As a result of these studies, some facial creams and lotions on the market contain kinetin as one of the active ingredients.

While most of these anti-aging studies focus on kinetin, all of the cytokinins that normally occur in coconut water seem to work together synergistically to produce anti-aging effects.[25] Coconut water contains among the highest concentration of cytokinins in the plant kingdom. These cytokinins have proven effective in retarding the processes that lead to premature aging and cellular breakdown in the skin, and there is now evidence that they may do the same for the eyes.

There is no medical cure for cataracts, and as we discussed earlier, the only medical solution is surgery to remove the natural lens and replace it with a synthetic one. A more natural approach is to alter the diet and increase the intake of antioxidant nutrients. While this will not cure cataracts, it has been shown to slow the progression of the disease and may even be helpful in preventing it, if started early in life, before the disease takes hold. Another approach that can enhance the effects of a nutritious diet is to increase blood ketone levels, with either a ketogenic or low-carb, coconut oil-based diet. The presence of ketones will greatly reduce lens exposure to free radicals and preserve antioxidant defenses. Another possible natural treatment that may be the best solution of all, is to bathe the eyes in coconut water.

Some years ago, one of my patients told me about a treatment for cataracts that she read about in a book by herbalist John Heinerman. He advised the patient to lie down and put several drops of fresh coconut water into the eyes, then apply a hot, damp washcloth over the eyes for about 10 minutes.

According to Heinerman, even one application is enough for significant improvement. My patient had cataracts, so she tried this approach on herself and happily reported that it worked. No more cataracts! I was surprised and a little skeptical at first, as I had never heard of coconut water for such a use before. I began researching the matter for myself, to learn more about the effects of coconut water on cataracts and health in general. In my research, I ran across an interesting incident that dramatically illustrates the potential benefit coconut water may have in treating cataract. This is Marjie's story, in her own words:

"We discovered this by accident while on a cruise ship (years ago). A few of us were on an island day trip and wanted to get off the beaten tourists' path, so we hired a bus and driver to take us to the opposite side of the island (only 10 of us on that big bus). A man and his wife were taking the cruise as a sort of last hoorah before her scheduled cataract surgery, we later found out. Anyway, there was a beautiful beach with coconuts lying everywhere and we got thirsty, but there was no drinking water. So we decided to open up some coconuts to quench our dry throats. We found a local with a big machete and through sign language we convinced him to open coconuts for us. The woman with the cataracts got splashed in one eye by the coconut juice, and it burned a bit. We were all digging through everything we had for something to relieve her eye 'injury.' All we came up with was one moist washcloth. Her husband wiped her eye and placed the washcloth over it. About 10 minutes later she announced we should head back to the ship. We did.

"The next morning, at breakfast, she said that her eye was much better and that she could see very well. We examined her eye closely and could not see any signs of the cataract, which was quite obvious the day before. She said she wished she had gotten splashed in both eyes. Then the idea dawned on us to 'splash' her other eye. We did that very day as soon as we got ashore and also repeated the other eye too. This time we were prepared. We went to the local market, grabbed a coconut, opened it, and strained it through a washcloth into a plastic cup, dribbled the juice into both eyes, placed a warm washcloth over both eyes, waited 10 minutes, and the rest is history. She went to her MD upon returning stateside—no cataracts and no surgery."

Stories like these don't prove that coconut water can cure cataracts, but they certainly suggest that it might be possible. To my knowledge, there has been no study that demonstrates that coconut water is useful for the treatment of cataracts; then again, no study has demonstrated that it cannot. This only means that, to date, there is no documented scientific proof.

While there may currently be little scientific evidence demonstrating the use of coconut water as a treatment for cataracts, there are ample studies that prove coconut water's potent antioxidant and anti-aging effects.[26-34] Putting coconut water in the eye does not cause any harm or discomfort, so there is no risk involved.

Since learning about this possible use for coconut water, I have mentioned it to people with cataracts. Interestingly, many of them have tried it and reported positive results, strongly suggesting that it really works, at least in some people. For example, Sandy H. successfully removed cataracts from both of her eyes with coconut water on two separate occasions. She treated only one eye at a time. She placed several drops of coconut water in her right eye using an eye dropper, let it sit for 3 to 5 minutes, then applied a warm, damp washcloth to the eye for about 10 minutes. She reported that the cataract was gone within a couple of hours. She only applied the coconut water once to achieve this remarkable result. Sandy waited a couple of weeks to see if the cataract would return, it didn't. Since her eye was clear and felt fine, she repeated the procedure on the left eye, with the same result.

Three years later, during a medical examination, the doctor told Sandy that her eyes were starting to develop cataracts again. She immediately knew what to do. Starting with the right eye, she repeated the procedure she had followed before; however, this time, she put the coconut water in an eye cup and soaked her eye for a minute or so. She then applied the warm, damp washcloth for about 10 minutes. Within 2 hours the cataract was gone. She waited a few days and repeated the procedure on the other eye with the identical result.

I have now heard from too many people who have cured themselves of cataracts using this method to say it is mere coincidence. Coincidences don't keep happening over and over again, especially with a condition that is generally considered irreversible.

Sandy was able to clear the cataracts in both eyes, twice. The reason why the cataracts came back after three years was probably because she made no significant changes to her diet or lifestyle during that time. The same conditions that initiated the cataracts in the first place remained and continued to work on her eyes after the initial treatment. If she would have improved her diet, including the addition of coconut oil, and made efforts to avoid those things that are known to be detrimental to good eye health, like certain drugs and food additives, her eyes may have remained clear for the rest of her life.

I suspect that for this procedure to work as well as reported, fresh coconut water from a real coconut is necessary. Nearly all the commercially available brands of coconut water sold in tetra pak containers, cans, and bottles are heat pasteurized. Some are even reconstituted from coconut water that has been boiled down into a syrup or powder. I don't know if this type of coconut water would have the same healing effect. The only commercially produced coconut water I would suggest trying in this situation, is a brand called Invo Coconut Water. This brand is not heat pasteurized. Invo uses a cold pasteurization process in which the water is subjected to a large amount of pressure at room temperature. This process guarantees the product is germ-free and essentially raw, just like fresh coconut water. You can tell it is different from other brands of commercially packaged coconut water because it tastes just like the water from a freshly opened coconut.

You can apply coconut water with an eye dropper or eye cup. I prefer an eye cup because the eyes are exposed to a greater amount of coconut water. The eye cup contains about ½ ounce (15 ml) of liquid. You place the cup up to your eye and tilt your head back, allowing the open eye to be bathed in the water. The process is repeated with the other eye. Follow this by lying down and applying a very warm, damp washcloth to the closed eye for about 10 minutes. Eye cups are available at most drug stores.

Fresh coconut water spoils quickly once it is removed from the coconut. You can keep it in a sealed container in the refrigerator for only a couple of days. Since you use only a small amount for your eyewash, you can drink the rest or freeze the remaining portion and use it later.

Since coconut water has a potentially huge effect on clearing cataracts, it may also have other benefits that are not as obvious, deeper within the eye. It is apparent that the water, or at least some of the antioxidant components in the water, are absorbed into the tissues. If they counter the runaway oxidation that is causing cataracts in the lens, then perhaps they can also do the same in other parts of eye. The coconut water eyewash may be a simple, effective method of clearing excessive oxidative stress from the retina and other parts of the eye.

Tissue degeneration resulting from oxidative stress is involved in many age-related eye diseases. Elevated intraocular pressure, a characteristic trait of glaucoma, may be caused by blockage in the fluid drainage canals of the eye. Much of the damage to the canals can be attributed to oxidative stress. Therefore, a treatment that could prevent the oxidative damage in the canals can potentially help prevent or treat glaucoma.[35] Coconut water may be able to provide that protection.

For maximum success, combine the use of coconut water with a nutritious low-carb diet rich in fresh vegetables, eggs, coconut oil, and other good foods. The lens of the eye contains and needs antioxidants to help protect it from oxidation and AGEs. Lutein and zeaxanthin are important antioxidants found in the lens, so your diet should include them. The lens also contains receptors for the neurotransmitter glutamate, which means it is highly susceptible to dietary MSG. MSG damages nerve tissues and causes severe oxidative stress that is harmful for the lens and can lead to cataracts.[36] Be careful with drugs as well, for many of them can cause cataracts. Antihistamines (allergy and cold medications) increase sensitivity to light and, consequently, increase risk of oxidation of the lens. The most widely used prescription drugs in the world, statins, can also cause cataracts. Using coconut water to heal cataracts may be fruitless if you are causing it at the same time with the use of drugs. Blood sugar levels also affect lens health, and you must get them under control if you want to be cataract-free.

As with any treatment, success will vary from person to person depending on a number of factors such as antioxidant status, blood sugar levels, and severity of the condition. Mild to moderate stages of cataracts will respond better than severe or advanced cases. If you don't see the improvement you expected after doing the coconut water wash, the problem may be due elevated blood sugar levels (from a high-carb diet), low antioxidant status, drug and tobacco use, eating the wrong types of fat, etc.

Prevention is always better than treatment. A simple preventive measure for cataracts—and, possibly, other age-related eye conditions—is to perform the coconut water eyewash periodically, I suggest every two to four weeks or so. If you would like to learn more about the effects of coconut water on eye health, its anti-aging effects, and its many other health properties, I recommend that you read my book *Coconut Water for Health and Healing.*

DRY EYE SYNDROME

Dry eye syndrome is probably the most common eye problem. As much as 48 percent of American adults have experienced this, at least to some degree. For some, it is only an occasional problem, while others endure it as a chronic condition. Dryness, scratchiness, red eyes, a burning sensation, and the feeling that a foreign object is in the eye are common symptoms. Forty-two percent of middle-aged women who have dry eye symptoms report blurred vision, and 43 percent of adults say they experience difficulty reading due to their symptoms.

Dry eye is caused by a lack of tears and affects the cornea and conjunctiva. Tears are essential for good eye health. They bathe the eye, washing out dust and debris and keep the eye moist and lubricated. They also contain enzymes that help prevent microorganisms from infecting the eye.

Tears consist of three essential components: water, oil, and mucous, each of which serves an important purpose. The watery portion keeps the eyes moist, the oil prevents evaporation and increases lubrication, and the mucous helps anchor the tears to the surface of eye. Each component is produced by a different gland. The watery part is produced by glands above the outer corner of the eyes. The oily part is produced by glands located in the eyelids, and the mucous is produced by cells in the conjunctiva.

Dry eye can occur due to a number of reasons including vitamin A deficiency, chronic dehydration, low-fat diet, blocked tear ducts, as a side effect of medications (antihistamines, antidepressants, certain blood pressure medicines, Parkinson's medications, birth control pills, and antiperspirants), and as a symptom of systemic disease such as lupus, rheumatoid arthritis, ocular rosacea, and Sjogren's syndrome.

The solution to the problem, in many cases, is relatively simple: make sure you consume enough vitamin A, that you are well hydrated (drink six to eight glasses of water a day), include ample good fats in your diet, and avoid troublesome medications. Medications are a major cause of dry eye syndrome. Many common over-the-counter drugs can cause it. If you use allergy medications or antiperspirants regularly, this can lead to chronic dry eye.

Many people have dry eye simply because they don't drink enough water. These people often rely on coffee or soda as their main source of fluids, but the body needs water. Chronic dehydration is a very common problem. A study done by researchers at Johns Hopkins Hospital in Baltimore discovered that up to 41 percent of the subjects they tested, both men and women ages 23 to 44, were chronically dehydrated. As we age, our sense of thirst decreases, rendering seniors more vulnerable to dehydration. Food surveys suggest that as much as 75 percent of the population, regardless of age, is chronically mildly dehydrated.

Coconut water is an excellent rehydration beverage, and absorbs into the bloodstream faster and more efficiently than water. People with dry eye find that it helps ease their symptoms. Below are some comments from people who suffer from dry eye syndrome.

"I have begun to drink 1 [serving of] coconut water a day and each day that I drink it, my eye drop usage drops dramatically! Seriously, I am much more comfortable and my eyes feel a million times better. I have been doing this over a month now and the change has been remarkable...I drink it first thing in the morning and it helps soooo much!!!"
–Gail

"Woke up with watery eyes today—awesome!...I've tried to hydrate with water before and did not have this happen."
–Deborah

"I've been trying different things to help with the dry eye, dry mouth, and sleeping through the night. I tried fish oil for several months, but nothing changed. I tried taking vitamin A, but no change. I drank a ton of water and it went right through me. I started drinking a huge glass of coconut water at night before bed and this has helped

tremendously…It doesn't make the problem go away completely, but it's been helping me make it through the night till morning."
–Jenny

"I've been drinking a cup or two a day for a week and have noticed an improvement in dryness. Actually two nights in a row now that I didn't feel the need to put gel in my eyes before bed and my eyes felt almost normal when waking up. This was huge for me, usually first thing I can't wait to put in my first drops of Restasis to try and get that normal feeling."
–Shari

"Have tried drinking coconut water directly from the fruit for the past 2 days—you are right, it does help with dry eyes! I asked the doctors about this as I am currently hospitalized, and they say that coconut water is even better than an IV for hydration, it balances the electrolytes and restores moisture where it is needed in the body. I am so happy about this discovery!"
–Dani

Drinking coconut water can help greatly when a person is dehydrated. If dehydration is not the cause for dry eye, then coconut water may not be the solution.

The most common treatment for dry eye is a medication known as ocular lubricant, or artificial tears, that helps to ease the dry, scratchy feeling. Depending on the severity of the condition, these eye drops may be used several times throughout the day to keep the eyes moist. However, ocular lubricants provide only temporary, incomplete relief, treating only the symptoms rather than any underlying condition.

It is now recognized that the primary cause of dry eye syndrome is a deficiency in the amount of oil secreted in the tears. Many people with dry eye syndrome can cry and shed tears, but the tears lack oil. Without an adequate amount of oil, the tears quickly evaporate, leaving the eyes dry. Since a lack of oil is a major cause, a possible simple solution is to add more fat into the diet, preferably coconut oil. Adding 2 to 3 tablespoons (30 to 45 ml) of coconut oil into the daily diet is of great help to many people with dry eyes.

We've been told to reduce our fat intake for so many years that some people have all but eliminated fat from their diets, but fat is an essential part of a nutritious diet. A fat deficiency can lead to dry skin and dry eyes. Simply adding more fat, and particularly coconut oil, into the diet can work wonders. "I told a friend about all of the supplements I'm taking for my dry eyes, and she was astounded," says Lidia. "She suggested that I stop taking the supplements and try coconut oil, 2 to 3 tablespoons a day, added in my food. I don't like taking so many supplements, so I decided to give it a try. I was amazed. It worked wonderfully and my skin has never felt so soft."

Charmian had a similar experience. For 2 years she had been having problems with itchy, irritated eyes that affected her sight so dramatically that it often made it impossible for her to drive. Her ophthalmologist said that she had lots of tears but they did not contain enough oil to properly lubricate her eye. He prescribed a special eyedrop solution for her, which helped. "About the same time I started with these drops," says Charmian, "I also started taking coconut oil daily. I used 2 to 3 tubes of the eyedrops and then realized I didn't need them anymore. I stopped using them for over 6 weeks. I didn't make the connection with the coconut oil until I ran out of the oil. On the fifth day without coconut oil I had to use the drops again. However, once I got back on my daily dose of coconut oil, I haven't needed them at all, and it has been over 3 months."

These changes are real, they don't happen simply because someone believes they are going to relieve their dry eyes. People have added coconut oil into their diets for other reasons totally unaware that it could have this effect. That is what happened to Katherine. "I have found that since I have been consuming 2 to 3 tablespoons of coconut oil each day, my eyes aren't dry anymore!" she says. "I began coconut oil for different reasons, and about 10 days into it, I noticed a few things: my brain fog has seriously diminished, and my eyes aren't dry or as tired anymore."

Another use of coconut oil is as an eyedrop solution—a natural alternative to artificial tears. People in the Caribbean use it this way to soothe irritated, dry eyes. Coconut oil can provide the eye with the missing layer of oil it needs to keep tears from evaporating too quickly. In addition, it can help calm inflammation, which has been identified as a major factor associated with dry eye.[37] Coconut oil can address this problem as well because of its anti-inflammatory properties.[38]

Just putting the oil around the eyes can help. "My mother has dry eyes, and has found relief by using coconut oil around her eyes at night," says Elaine. "She was initially using it just for a night cream/moisturizer effect, but found that her eyes felt much better within a few days."

Putting the oil directly into the eyes is even better. It is completely harmless and does not sting or hurt the eyes in any way, but it can trigger a temporary increase in tears. Melt some coconut oil and put it into an eye dropper bottle. Whenever you want to use the oil make sure it is in its liquid form. If not, gently heat the bottle in hot water or on the warmer of your stovetop. Once it is melted, make sure it is not too hot, and put a couple of drops into each eye. It is also good for washing out debris and irritants.

Coconut oil eyedrops can be used with standard medications. In fact, adding coconut oil helps relieve the irritating side effects often associated with ocular lubricants. "I have been experimenting with raw coconut oil for a few months," says Taran, "and I have found that it helps me with side effects from the drops. My eyes are not as red and irritated when I use it compared to when I don't. I have tried doing it in just one eye and the difference is very clear to me; irritation, itching, and redness in one eye but not the other."

Coconut oil eyedrops are also beneficial for washing out dust and irritants or whenever the eyes seem to burn or sting, whatever the cause. "Sometimes my eyes become very irritated and burn," says Jason. "I don't know why this happens but coconut oil has brought me relief. I discovered this after several days of torment. I thought that maybe putting coconut oil in my eyes would help. I have had great success using it on my skin and I had heard of others using it in their eyes, so I gave it a try. I wanted my eyes to be in contact with the oil for as long as possible, so I put a few drops into each eye just before going to bed. My eyes felt greatly improved the next day. I followed the same procedure the following night just to make sure that whatever was bothering my eyes would not return. It worked. Some months later my eyes started to become irritated just like they had before, so I applied the coconut oil eyedrops and they cleared right up. I don't know what the oil does, but it works."

"I have used coconut oil in my dry eyes," says Carol, "and have found it to be the best solution to dryness and also blepharitis (inflammation of the eyelids)...Right now I heat a small amount of oil and put it in my eyes before bed. I wake up without crusty eyes and my eyes are not dry like they are with conventional drops."

The best approach to dry eye syndrome is to add an adequate amount of coconut oil into the diet and use coconut oil eyedrops as needed.

Many common over-the-counter drugs can lead to dry eyes, most notably antihistamines and decongestants such as Benadryl, Contac, Nyquil, Sinutab, Dimetapp, Dristan, and others. These drugs are used specifically to dry out the sinuses, but they also dry the eyes and can cause dehydration. The artificial sweetener aspartame (NutriSweet), which is used in hundreds of products, is also known to cause dry eyes. If you drink sugar-free soda, it most likely is sweetened with aspartame.

Another common cause of dry eye is underarm antiperspirants. Not only do these dry out the sweat glands, but they also dry the eyes and mouth. "I don't normally use antiperspirants," says Jim, "but I was going to give an important presentation and I was nervous, so I

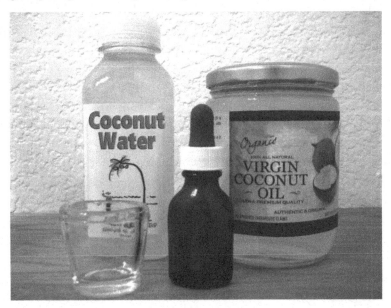

Coconut water can be administered to the eyes using an eye cup or eye dropper. Coconut oil is best delivered with an eye dropper.

sprayed it on, a good double dose because when I get nervous, I sweat a lot. It worked a little too well, in fact. I didn't sweat all that evening or the all the next day. It dried me up terribly. My eyes and mouth were extremely dry. The effects lasted for about two days."

EYE INFECTIONS
(CONJUNCTIVITIS, BLEPHARITIS, AND STYE)

Coconut oil possesses antimicrobial properties that can aid in preventing and treating mild eye infections and reduce inflammation. The medium chain fatty acids in coconut oil have been shown to be effective in killing many common forms of bacteria, viruses, and fungi, including Candida, a frequent inhabitant of the skin and mucous membranes and a potential source of infection. Coconut oil works wonders when applied topically on the skin, soothing irritation and calming inflammation. It has proven to be an effective treatment for many common skin infections including ringworm, athlete's foot, nail fungus, and diaper rash. Interestingly, the fatty acids in coconut oil are deadly to potentially harmful microorganisms, yet they are harmless to our cells. In fact, our cells absorb these medium chain fatty acids and use them as food. To germs they are deadly, but to us they are nourishment.

Coconut oil can do the same for the eyes. Coconut oil or MCTs are used in a number of commercially available medicated eyedrop solutions to treat infections and inflammation.[39-40] In these commercial products, MCTs are combined with medications to enhance the effects of the product; however, coconut oil alone can be used to treat mild eye infections.

Various forms of bacteria can infect the conjunctiva and cause conjunctivitis. Conjunctivitis causes the sclera to turn red or pink and become irritated and weepy. Blepharitis can be caused by a bacterial or fungal infection of the tiny glands and hair follicles on the surface of the eyelids. It causes the eyelids to become red and swollen. A stye is a bacterial infection in one of the small glands on the edges of the eyelids or just under the eyelids. A stye is small and looks like a pimple on the eyelid, which is basically what it is. Styes can be somewhat painful, and both children and adults can get styes from rubbing their eyes with dirty hands.

How to Apply Eyedrops

To properly apply eyedrops, follow these steps:

- Wash your hands.
- Tilt your head back.
- Hold the eyedropper in one hand and bring it as close as possible to your eye.
- Using your free hand, pull down your lower eyelid to form a pocket.
- To keep from blinking, look up and away from the dropper tip just before you release the drop.
- Place 1 to 2 drops into the lower eyelid pocket. The volume of 2 drops exceeds the capacity that can cover the surface of the eye, so there is no need to use additional drops.
- Release the eyelid, close your eye, and keep it closed for 1 to 2 minutes. This keeps the drop in the eye and helps prevent it from draining into the tear duct. Do not squeeze the eye shut or rub it. You can also press your finger to the inside corner of the eye, on the tear duct, to keep the oil from leaking out.

Coconut oil eyedrops applied two to three times a day can be a quick and simple solution for most infections. However, if an infection persists for more than a couple of days with the use of coconut oil, a stronger antibacterial may be needed. Check with your doctor, because a serious infection may cause permanent damage.

SJOGREN'S SYNDROME

After winning her first-round match during the 2011 U.S. Open, 31-year old tennis star Venus Williams unexpectedly withdrew from the competition. Williams, a former Wimbledon champion and seven-time Olympic gold medalist, had been struggling physically following her recent diagnosis of Sjogren's syndrome. Her diagnosis brought the relatively little-known disease to public awareness.

Sjogren's (pronounced *show-grins*) syndrome is an autoimmune disorder that affects as many as 4 million people in the United States. Most who develop this condition are older than forty at the time of diagnosis. Women are nine times more likely to develop Sjogren's syndrome than men. The primary symptoms are excessively dry eyes and mouth. Other common symptoms may include fatigue, dental cavities (caused by lack of saliva), difficulty swallowing or chewing, hoarseness, changes in the sense of taste, blurred vision, sensitivity to light, corneal ulcers, skin rash, dry skin, dry cough, vaginal dryness, oral yeast infections (thrush), and joint or muscle pain. Arthritis is common in Sjogren's patients. Like other autoimmune disorders, Sjogren's is accompanied by chronic inflammation.

Doctors don't know what causes Sjogren's syndrome, and there is no known cure. Treatment consists of easing symptoms of dryness with artificial tears and saliva products, along with nonsteroidal anti-inflammatory drugs and other medications.

People with Sjogren's syndrome are finding that coconut oil offers a great deal of relief from their symptoms. "I was diagnosed with Sjogren's syndrome three years ago," says CJ. "I was taking prescriptions for a number of secondary conditions associated with Sjogren's. After much research and experimentation, I changed the way I eat. My diet now is mostly low-carb and grain-free, with lots of water to stay hydrated. I eat coconut and cook everything in coconut oil. The new diet, along with coconut oil, has been a lifesaver. I've been able to get completely off all my medications. I feel so much better now."

Conrado Dayrit, MD, tells of a colleague who developed Sjogren's later in life. "He was my classmate in medical school and he had attended our class reunions. We celebrated our silver, then our golden and diamond anniversaries, but then he stopped coming. He was sick. His mouth had little saliva; he could not swallow without drinking water. His eyes were smarting and he needed artificial tears every hour or two to moisten the dry conjunctiva. His skin was dry and cracking. Worst of all, his anorectal passage was dry and moving his bowels was torture. He lost much weight. He consulted various specialists. Being a doctor himself, he had to agree with the diagnosis of Sjogren's syndrome. He read medical textbooks, combed the literature and the Internet seeking newer therapies. The prognosis was gloomy, the recommended treatment unsatisfactory. Fortunately, he did not suffer any complications like arthritis, lupus, nephritis, or thromboangitis, but he was miserable. We learned about his illness when he forced himself to attend one class reunion. I suggested that he try taking four tablespoons daily of virgin coconut oil. He followed my advice. Two months later, he reported to me by phone that he was 70 to 80 percent improved! He could eat and move his bowels normally. His skin had regained its elasticity. His eyes needed no more than two or three drops a day. He had gained back his strength, energy, and wellbeing. All this just with virgin coconut oil and no drugs... Virgin coconut oil is the only treatment so far that has shown such dramatic effect as this."[41]

How coconut oil is able to help those with Sjogren's syndrome is yet to be determined, but it is probably due to some combination of the oil's anti-inflammatory, antimicrobial, immune-regulating, and nutritional properties.

It is apparent that consuming coconut oil can have a positive effect on Sjogren's syndrome. Some people have reported remarkable benefits by simply swishing it in their mouths—a process known as oil pulling. "I have been oil pulling with coconut oil for a month," says Velta M. "Already, I have seen so many improvements in my health. I have Sjogren's syndrome with dry eyes, dry mouth, and fatigue. Sores in [my] mouth are gone, eye specialist said my eyes are better than they have been in three years, my sinuses are clearer, I am sleeping better, way better energy—and I am able to yawn widely, which I have not been able to do for years because of TMJ. It is truly miraculous!"

The evidence showing that coconut oil, taken internally or used in oil pulling, can help treat Sjogren's syndrome doesn't come entirely from testimonials from doctors and patients. A pilot study conducted by Dr. Leslie Laing, PhD, DDS, an assistant professor of dentistry at the University of Toronto, showed similar results when Sjogren's patients used coconut oil for oil pulling.

"Since my primary research is with the autoimmune disorder of Sjogren's Syndrome (SS)," says Laing, "I'm on the lookout for methods to increase either salivary flow or to moisturize the mouth of those afflicted with SS, which affects up to 430,000 post-menopausal Canadian women." The problem can be so bad that some people wake up having to "peel their cheeks off their teeth," Laing says. "I thought oil pulling might at least provide lubrication for their mouths. The emerging evidence in the literature that such a safe product might also inhibit bacteria associated with cavities gave me the idea that this might be worth investigating."

Before embarking on her pilot study, Dr. Laing tested the procedure on herself and her two sons for several weeks. "I found that the oil had not only a pleasant taste but also lubricated the mouth. Even my dogs like the virgin coconut oil!" she says. Most dogs love the taste of coconut oil and it cleans and whitens their teeth and eliminates bad doggy breath too.

"The technique itself caused stimulation of saliva production, at least in me, and I ended up with a lot more liquid in my mouth after 15 minutes of oil pulling than when I had started! I reasoned that the sheer mechanics of the technique may have a stimulating effect on saliva production in SS patients."

Encouraged by the results, Laing had a dozen of her Sjogren's patients, in addition to others who had xerostomia (dry mouth) due to other causes, try oil pulling. The subjects oil pulled with virgin coconut oil for 20 minutes every day for three weeks. She measured their bacterial and fungal loads before and after the study. When the results came in, Laing was astounded.

The subjects were pleased with the effect, stating that their mouths felt more comfortable after the oil pulling and that they didn't have to interrupt their sleep at night to get a drink of water.

"Not only did they find their mouths felt a lot moister, they also noticed that whatever teeth they had left—because they might have been decayed—they looked brighter," Laing said. "There seemed to be a glossiness to them, which they wouldn't have had with a dry mouth."

Amazingly, bacterial counts decreased in some of the subjects by as much as tenfold. Laing found reductions in the two major bacteria species that cause dental cavities and reduced levels of yeast (Candida), which can cause oral thrush. Reducing these yeast levels can help with bloating, gas, diarrhea, constipation, fatigue, headaches and even depression. "These were very encouraging results," says Laing.[42]

Dr. Laing plans to repeat the pilot study with more patients to confirm her results, but for now she says oil pulling has clear antibacterial benefits and appears to offer hope to Sjogren's sufferers. "I'm not making claims that this is a be-all and end-all. These are preliminary results, but I am liking what I'm seeing," she says.

There is also evidence that improved blood sugar control and ketones can help prevent and possibly reduce the symptoms of Sjogren's. Calorie restriction, which has been shown to moderate blood sugar and increase blood ketones, has proven effective in reducing the severity of the symptoms associated with the disease.[43]

Coconut oil is harmless, even in relatively large doses. If you suffer from Sjogren's it won't hurt to try it, and it may do a whole lot of good. Adding the oil into a low-carb diet is the most effective approach to address this condition, but using the oil in the eyes or as a mouthwash as part of your daily oral hygiene routine may enhance the effects.

ARE YOU AT RISK?

Degenerative eye disorders often arise without any warning. They develop so gradually that before you notice anything is amiss, substantial damage may have already occurred. Once the damage is done, it can be very difficult, if not impossible, to correct completely. Regular eye examines will help to spot potential problems. However, your optometrist may not identify the problem in the early stages either. Currently there are no medical tests or procedures that can identify individuals who are at high risk for visual difficulties. It is only after damage has occurred and some level of vision loss is present can doctors can identify a problem exists and make a diagnosis.

Fortunately, there are ways you can determine your risk right now, long before obvious signs or symptoms arise. You can do this mostly on your own, without the use of invasive medical procedures. First, evaluate your diet. If you are eating a diet loaded with sugar, refined carbohydrates, processed vegetable oils, and food additives (aspartame, MSG, etc.), your risk is high. Second, get your fasting blood sugar measured. If your fasting blood sugar level is 101 mg/dl (5.6 mmol/l) or more, your risk is high, and if it is 126 mg/dl (7 mmol/l) or higher, your risk is very high. Another measure of blood sugar is the A1C test. If your A1C measures 5.7 or greater, you are at high risk. Third, check the drugs you are taking and see if they might affect vision. The longer you take suspect drugs, the greater your risk. Tobacco use also greatly increases risk of all the major eye disorders.

The solution is obvious, change your diet, lower your blood sugar levels, and discontinue all unnecessary drugs. The way to do this is described in Chapter 11. Simply improving your diet, as described in Chapter 11, will lower your blood sugar levels and improve overall health, eliminating the need for most drugs. Not only will your risk of eye disorders decrease, but all aspects of your health will improve.

11

The Low-Carbohydrate Diet

LOW-CARB PROGRAM FOR BETTER EYE HEALTH

Insulin resistance appears to be a common problem in all forms of neurodegeneration. Improvement can occur when blood sugar is brought under control. Therefore, blood sugar control is vital in the treatment of degenerative eye conditions.

The only way to compensate for insulin resistance is to control blood glucose levels. This is accomplished by restricting the amount of carbohydrate consumed. Prior to the discovery of insulin in the 1920s, a low-carb diet consisting of 75 percent fat, 17 percent protein, and 8 percent carbohydrate was used successfully in the treatment of diabetes. The problem with this diet, as well as the classic ketogenic diet (90 percent fat, 8 percent protein, and 2 percent carbohydrate), is that it is too difficult for most people to adhere to for any length of time. Fortunately, such a strict diet isn't necessary in order to limit carbohydrate consumption or boost ketone levels. A less strict high-fat, low-carbohydrate diet has shown to provide a similar degree of protection, while allowing a much greater variety of foods and even a higher, yet still restricted, intake of carbohydrate.

The dietary approach proposed in this book combines a low-carb diet with the ketone-producing, brain-protecting power of MCTs from coconut oil. This dietary program produces enough ketones to supply the brain and eyes with the fuel they need to function properly. In addition, it enhances insulin sensitivity, normalizes metabolic parameters, calms inflammation, and stops runaway oxidative stress and destructive glycation. In other words, it removes many of the underlying factors that lead to neurodegeneration and provides the energy and building materials needed for eye revitalization.

This book is written just as much for the person who is concerned about his or her future eye health as it is for those who are already experiencing problems. Taking care of your eyes starting now, before symptoms surface, is your best insurance that you will retain good vision long into old age.

I offer two approaches to the diet. The first is designed for prevention. This diet is suitable for those who have normal or close to normal fasting blood sugar levels (below 91 mg/dL) and have no symptoms of age-related eye disorders. This diet is designed to be very simple and easy to follow and allow a generous degree of freedom in food choices so it can be easily maintained for life.

The second approach is for those who are already experiencing age-related eye problems and need a more intense program to stop the progression of the condition and provide the body with the opportunity to heal itself. There are two levels to this treatment diet: one for those with severe insulin resistance and would be classified as diabetic, and the other for those with less severe insulin resistance, who would fit in the pre-diabetic stage.

Low-Carb Prevention Diet

The prevention diet is purposely designed to be as easy as possible and to allow ample freedom of food choices, while still restricting carbohydrate intake and improving insulin sensitivity. You don't have to worry about counting calories, grams of carbohydrate, or measuring or weighing food. The primary approach to this diet is to limit foods containing the highest amount of carbohydrate, which cause the most problems.

The foods with the richest carbohydrate content are grains, legumes, and potatoes. Of these, grains are the biggest problem, primarily because they are so pervasive in our diet. Simply eliminating grains can have a major impact on blood sugar control. Frankly, all grains should be removed from the diet. Also excluded are flours made from these grains, including their products, such as bread, tortillas, chips, and pasta. Legumes and potatoes should be limited to just small portions, a half-cup or so periodically, if any at all.

Another major source of carbohydrate that is often eaten with grains is sugar. All sugars contain basically the same amount of carbohydrate regardless of their source or method of processing. So-called natural sweeteners like dehydrated sugarcane juice, date sugar, molasses, maple syrup, and honey are just as rich in carbs as white table sugar, so these should be avoided, as should all candy, desserts, sodas, and fruit juice.

Fruit can also be a high source of carbohydrates. While you don't need to eliminate all fruit, it should be consumed in moderation. Avoid dried fruits because removing the water content concentrates the sugar and intensifies the sweetness and carb content.

Does all this mean you can't eat a little cake or a slice of bread occasionally? It's best you don't, but the diet is flexible enough that small portions, such as one slice of bread, can be consumed on special occasions, though definitely not every day or every other day and ideally not at all.

Instead of eating breads and baked goods, eat more freshly prepared vegetables. These are excellent sources of essential vitamins, minerals, and antioxidants that are so important to eye health. Starchy vegetables, such as potatoes and beans, should be replaced for the most part by lower-carb vegetables like cauliflower, broccoli, asparagus, spinach, and such.

Meat, fish, and eggs contain such small amounts of carbohydrate that you don't need to worry about how much you eat. However, be aware that many prepared meats, like cold cuts and ham, normally contain sugar and often MSG, so it is best to eat fresh meats. The carb content of dairy varies. Butter, cream, and hard cheeses are low in carbs; milk is a moderate source; and sweetened dairy, like yogurt and ice cream, are high in carbs. Choose low-carb dairy products over the high-carb options.

In addition to the low-carb diet, for prevention you should consume at least 1 to 3 tablespoons (15 to 45 ml) of coconut oil daily. The oil can be used in cooking or meal preparation or added to the food afterward. For example, you can add a spoonful of coconut oil to a bowl of soup, in a casserole, or on top of cooked vegetables.

Low-Carb Treatment Diets

There are two treatment options based on fasting blood sugar levels. The purpose of these diets is to reduce these levels and to increase blood ketone levels. Each diet has assigned to it a total daily carbohydrate consumption limit in grams that needs to be strictly followed, as described below:

Low-Carb 25 Gram Diet

If fasting blood glucose is 126 mg/dl (7 mmol/l) or greater, carbohydrate consumption is limited to a maximum of 25 grams per day. No single meal should exceed half the daily total carbohydrate allowance (12.5 grams). In addition, consume 4 to 5 tablespoons (60 to 74 ml) of coconut oil daily.

Low-Carb 50 Gram Diet

If fasting blood glucose is 101 to 125 mg/dl (5.6 to 6.9 mmol/l), carbohydrate consumption is limited to a maximum of 50 grams per day. No single meal should exceed half the daily total carbohydrate allowance (25 grams). In addition, consume 4 to 5 tablespoons (60 to 74 ml) of coconut oil daily.

Both of these diets are ketogenic; that is, they will trigger the conversion of stored body fat into ketones and raise blood ketone levels. The Low-Carb 25 Gram Diet will elevate blood ketones higher than the Low-Carb 50 Gram Diet. The 50 gram diet is a mild ketogenic diet and in some people ketone levels will show minimal measurable increase, if any. Ketone levels are boosted by the consumption of between 4 to 5 tablespoons of coconut oil per day, which is recommended for each of these diets. The combination of a very low-carb diet with this amount of coconut oil can raise blood ketones to therapeutic levels.

The tablespoon referred to here is not the same as the tablespoon commonly used for eating. A tablespoon is a unit of measurement that equals 14.8 ml of liquid, or for ease of calculation 15 ml. Four tablespoons is equivalent to 60 ml; 5 tablespoons makes 74 ml. You may add additional fats and oils to the diet, such as butter or red palm oil. Don't be concerned about the fat causing you to gain weight, because it won't. When combined with a low-carb diet, fat satisfies hunger so you will tend to eat less, and you may actually end up losing weight. If you want to learn more about how a low-carb, coconut oil based diet can help you lose weight, I recommend you read my book *The Coconut Ketogenic Diet.*

Don't try to consume all the coconut oil at one time or try taking it by the spoonful. The coconut oil should be mixed with food and spread throughout the day, consuming some at each meal. Prepare your food with the oil, and add some to your food before eating.

We have been told to avoid fat for so many years that many people are not accustomed to eating a healthy proportion of fat in their meals. Some have avoided fat for so long that they are unable to properly digest any added fat, and if those people add 4 to 5 tablespoons of any oil to the diet, they may experience some degree of intestinal cramping or diarrhea. For this reason, I recommend that you add the coconut oil into your diet slowly, over a period of several weeks or months. This will allow time for your digestive system to adjust to the increased fat intake. Start off by adding only 1 tablespoon (15 ml) of coconut oil into your diet. This is added fat and not total fat. If you experience no problems with 1 tablespoon a day, boost it to 2 tablespoons daily, and gradually add more until you reach 4 to 5 tablespoons. If you experience undesirable digestive symptoms, back off on the oil by 1 or ½ tablespoon. If you have no problems at this level, stay there for a few weeks, and then try adding 1 or ½ tablespoon.

Some people can add 4 to 5 tablespoons of coconut oil into their daily diet immediately without any problem. Others may not be able to tolerate more than 1 tablespoon a day at first. Over time, though, you should be able to handle larger amounts of fat. Most people can work up to 4 to 5 tablespoons of added coconut oil daily within a month or two.

I recommend that people remain on each diet indefinitely, depending on their fasting blood sugar levels. If your blood sugar level is 126 mg/dl (7 mmol/l) or more, stay on the Low-Carb 25 Gram Diet. If you are able to reduce your fasting blood sugar to within 101-125 mg/dl (5.6 to 6.9 mmol/l), then you can adopt the Low-Carb 50 Gram Diet. If you are able to reduce your fasting blood sugar to 100 mg/dl (5.5 mmol/l) or lower, you can follow the Low-Carb Prevention Diet, which is also suitable as a maintenance diet.

BASIC GUIDELINES FOR THE LOW-CARB DIET

The low-carb diet accomplishes many things. In addition to the benefits mentioned in previous chapters, this diet will condition your body to burn fat in place of sugar; change destructive eating patterns; stop uncontrollable food cravings; break addictions to sugar, soda, caffeine, white bread, and other junk foods; allow you to enjoy eating full-fat and full-flavored foods without guilt; let you experience the delicious taste of whole, natural foods; change your frame of mind about foods; stabilize blood sugar; allow your body a chance to heal; relinquish your dependence on many medications; and enjoy life to a greater extent.

Depending on your fasting blood sugar readings, you will follow the Prevention Diet or the 25 or 50 Gram diets. You do not need to count calories, measure the amount of fat or protein consumed, or limit what you eat, except for carbohydrate. Eat until you are satisfied but not stuffed, as overeating reduces the effectiveness of the diet. As much as 58 percent of the protein you eat can be converted into glucose, so you do not want to over-consume high-protein foods either, but you are encouraged to eat lots of vegetables. Since fat produces very little glucose, you can eat as much as you desire.

A person can live on any of these, including the 25 Gram diet, indefinitely, as none of these diets are lacking in nutrients and provide plenty of nutrition for optimal health. Considering that you will be replacing the breads and grains with nutritious vegetables, it will probably a far healthier diet than you have ever eaten in your life.

With the treatment diets, you must calculate every gram of carbohydrate you eat. This is important. As you gain experience, you will be able to prepare meals without actually calculating each gram of carbohydrate. But for the first few months you need to pay particular attention to stay within your carbohydrate limit.

Most fresh meats, fish, fowl, and all fats contain little to no carbohydrate. Eggs, cheese, and lettuce contain very small amounts. Use the Net Carbohydrate Counter in the appendix to calculate the amount of net carbohydrate in your meals. The term "net carbohydrate" refers to carbohydrate that is digestible, provides calories, and raises blood sugar. Dietary fiber is also a carbohydrate, but it does not raise blood sugar or supply calories, so it is not included. Most plant foods contain both digestible carbohydrate, as well as fiber. To calculate the net carbohydrate content, subtract the fiber from the total. The Carbohydrate Counter in the appendix lists net carbohydrate on various whole foods. You can figure out the net carbohydrate content of packaged foods yourself, as the Nutrition Facts label on the packaging shows the amount of calories, fat, carbohydrate, protein, and other nutrients per serving. Under the "Total Carbohydrate" heading you will see "Dietary Fiber." To calculate the net carbohydrate content, subtract the grams of fiber listed from the grams of total carbohydrate.

The Carbohydrate Counter lists the most common vegetables, fruits, dairy, grains, nuts, and seeds. To find foods not on the list, including many popular packaged and restaurant foods, go online to www.calorieking.com; this website will provide you with a list of everything that is included on the nutrition labels of various foods. To find the net carbohydrate content, you must go through the same steps, subtract the fiber from total carbohydrate listed. Several websites provide the carbohydrate count on various foods, some others are www.carb-counter.org and www.cocoketodiet.com.

In order to stay under your carbohydrate limit for the day, you will want to eliminate or dramatically reduce all high-carb foods. For instance, a slice of white bread contains 12 grams of carbohydrate. If you are on the Low-Carb 25 Gram Diet, just two slices will bring you to your day's limit. Since all vegetables and fruits contain carbohydrate, you would be restricted to eating only meat and fat for the rest of the day in order to stay under your 25 gram limit—which is not a good idea. A single medium-size baked potato contains 33 grams of carbohydrate—more than a day's allotment. An apple has 18 grams, an orange has 12, and a medium-size banana 24. Breads and grains contain the highest amount of carbohydrate. A single 4-inch pancake without any syrup or sweeteners has 13 grams, a 10-inch tortilla has 34 grams, and a plain 4½-inch bagel has 57. Candy and desserts are even higher in carbohydrate and provide almost no nutritional value, so they should be completely eliminated from the diet. All breads and grains should be eliminated on the 25 gram diet.

Vegetables, however, have a much lower carbohydrate content. One cup of asparagus or raw cabbage has 2 grams, and a cup of cauliflower has 3. All types of lettuce are very low in carbohydrate; a cup of shredded lettuce has only about 0.6 gram. You can easily fill up on green salad and other low-carb vegetables without worrying too much about going over your carbohydrate limit.

Even on the Low-Carb 25 Gram Diet a limited amount of fruit can be consumed. Fruits with the lowest carbohydrate content are berries such as blackberries (½ cup 3.5 grams), boysenberries (½ cup 4.5 grams), raspberries (½ cup 3 grams), and strawberries (½ cup, sliced 4.8 grams). Any fruit, vegetable, or even grain product can be eaten, as long as the portion is not so large that it puts you over your carbohydrate limit. Since most fruits, starchy vegetables, and breads are high in carbohydrate, it is best to simply avoid them altogether.

Let's look at a typical daily meal plan for the Low-Carb 25 Gram Diet. Net carbs for each item are listed in parentheses.

Breakfast

Omelet with 2 eggs (1 g), 1 ounce of cheddar cheese (0.5 g), ½ cup sliced mushrooms (1 g), 2 ounces of diced sugar-free ham (0 g), and one teaspoon of chopped chives (0 g), cooked in 1 tablespoon of coconut oil (0 g). Net carbohydrate count 2.5 grams.

Lunch

Tossed green salad with 2 cups shredded lettuce (1 g), ½ cup shredded carrot (4 g), ¼ cup diced sweet bell pepper (1 g), ½ medium tomato (2 g), ¼ avocado (0 g), ½ cup shredded cabbage (1 g), 3 ounces chopped roasted chicken (0 g), 1 tablespoon roasted sunflower seeds (1 g), topped with 2 tablespoons of olive oil-based Italian dressing, without sugar (1 g). Net carbohydrate count 12 grams.

Dinner

One pork chop (0 g), cooked in 1 tablespoon coconut oil (0 g), 4 spears cooked asparagus (2 g), with 1 teaspoon butter (0 g), 2 cups cooked cauliflower (3 g) topped with 1 ounce of Colby cheese (0.5 g) with various herbs and spices (0 g) to enhance flavor. Net carbohydrate count 5.5 grams.

Total net carbohydrate consumed in the above three meals is 20 grams, which is 5 grams under the daily limit. As you can see from this example, the diet provides a variety of nutritious foods. In a Low-Carb 50 Gram Diet, 30 grams of net carbs could be added to the above.

A Low-Carb Prevention Diet is very lenient in comparison to the other two diets. It essentially includes all types of foods. Simply reducing portion sizes or frequency of eating starchy vegetables, fruits, grain products, and even occasional treats can easily keep total carbohydrate consumption within bounds.

For comparison, let's look at the carbohydrate content of some typical unrestricted meals. A typical breakfast might include a 1 cup serving of Frosted Flakes cereal (35 g) with ½ cup serving of 2% milk (12.5 g). Total carbohydrate count comes to 47 grams. A single serving of this cold cereal, which is very typical in carb content, exceeds the 25 gram limit and eats up almost the entire carbohydrate allotment of the 50 gram limit. Obviously, cold cereals are not a good option for those following a low-carb eating plan.

Most people realize that cold breakfast cereals are not the healthiest of foods. People eat them because they are convenient, quick, and generally tasty. They certainly shouldn't eat them for their nutritional content, no matter how healthy they claim to be. Hot, whole grain cereal is considered a better choice. While a bowl of hot oatmeal is more nutritious than an equal portion of cold cereal, the carbohydrate content is about the same. A one cup serving of cooked oatmeal (21.3 g), with 1 tablespoon of sugar (12 g) and ½ cup of 2% milk (12.5 g) provides a total carbohydrate count of 45.8 grams.

A typical lunch might include a McDonald's Big Mac hamburger (42 g), one medium fries (43.3 g), and a 12-ounce soda (39.9 g), providing a whopping 125.2 grams of carbohydrate, far more than the daily limit of the diet programs.

A typical dinner might include three medium-sized slices of pepperoni pizza (97.2 g) and a 12-ounce soda (39.9 g), providing 137.1 grams of carbohydrate.

Most typical meals are carbohydrate-rich. Consequently, the average American, European, or Australian consumes approximately 300 grams of carbohydrate a day. The best way to avoid excess carbohydrate is to make your meals at home using fresh, low-carb ingredients.

Does this mean you can't have pizza anymore? You will have to make some difficult decisions. Do you want pizza or would you prefer to avoid age-related visual problems? The choice is yours. You must decide if eating pizza is more important to you than your ability to see clearly as you age. If you think eating pizza, ice cream, or soda won't hurt you, it is likely that you are addicted to those foods. You are in denial, and a sure sign of addiction is to ignore sound reason in favor of satisfying cravings. You need this diet to break those addictions.

This low-carb eating plan really doesn't forbid any type of food, it only sets limits on how much you eat. So, while you can eat pizza occasionally, you must restrict the portion size and make adjustments in the other foods you eat so your daily carbohydrates consumption remains within the limits established by your diet program.

It is not a good idea to be too indulgent by eating one high-carb meal in anticipation of eliminating all carbs from the other two meals to make up for it. Let's assume you are on the Low-Carb 50 Gram Diet and you splurge by eating a piece of pie with 46 grams of carbohydrate. That leaves you with just 4 grams of carbs for the rest of the day. You would have to eat almost nothing but meat for two meals to make up for it. Even if you manage to do this, it is not a good idea. The 46 grams of carbohydrate consumed all at once will unleash a metabolic tidal wave in your body. The reason for limiting carbohydrate consumption in the first place is to avoid large influxes of sugar into your bloodstream, as this is what throws the body out of whack. It is best to divide your carbohydrate consumption over all three meals so no single meal contains more than half of the total daily allotment.

Obviously, you should not gorge yourself on pizza or ice cream as you may have as a teenager. The body is very sensitive to carbohydrates. A single candy bar can be very destructive, for the sugar it contains is enough to block the formation of ketone bodies and significantly lower ketone levels, not to mention what it does to blood sugar levels.

Food preferences can and do change. As you begin to eat more vegetables, especially when combined with butter, cheese, and rich sauces, they will become more satisfying than the junk foods you used to eat.

You are encouraged to eat at least one fresh, raw salad every day. A variety of tossed green salads can be made by simply changing the type of vegetables, toppings, and dressings you use.

Homemade salad dressings are generally best. If you use store bought dressing, avoid those with added sugar, and check the Nutrition Facts labels for carbohydrate content.

Very simple dinners may consist of a main course of your favorite meat—roast beef, roasted chicken, lamb chop, baked salmon, lobster, or whatever—served with a side dish or two of raw or cooked vegetables, such as steamed broccoli topped with butter and melted cheddar cheese.

The popularization of low-carb dieting in recent years has fueled an explosion of low-carb recipes and cookbooks. Many hundreds of low-carb recipes can be found on the Internet, freely accessible to all. Just be sure to check the total carbohydrate content, for not all recipes that claim to be low-carb are really that low. Many reduced-carb versions of standard favorites still deliver a substantial amount of carbohydrate. Keep in mind that just because a recipe may be low-carb, that does not make it ketogenic. The vast majority of low-carb recipes are not ketogenic. Because it can be difficult to find truly ketogenic recipes that also taste good, I have compiled a book of all my favorite ketogenic recipes titled the *Dr. Fife's Keto Cookery*. Each recipe includes the precise number of grams of fat, carbohydrate, and protein for each serving, so you know exactly what you are eating. Since cooking the keto way can be a challenge for many people, especially at first, this book can be an invaluable tool.

On your journey into the world of ketogenic eating, you are encouraged to eat full-fat foods, butter, cream, coconut oil, the fat on meat, and chicken skin. Fat is good for you! It satisfies hunger and prevents food cravings, and your desire for sweets will greatly diminish. Because fat is filling, hunger will be satisfied with less food, so total calorie consumption may decline somewhat. Those who are overweight may even see a reduction in weight. Underweight and undernourished people usually don't have a problem with losing weight, but the added fat in the diet will help them reach a healthier body weight.

Eating out can be a little challenging, but it has gotten much easier over the years. Because of the popularity of low-carbing, many restaurants now offer low-carb options. Most every restaurant that sells hamburgers, including all the popular fast food restaurants, offer bunless hamburgers. These hamburgers include everything you would expect in a regular hamburger but are wrapped in a blanket of lettuce without the bun. Even if this item isn't listed on the menu, most restaurants will be happy to make it for you on request.

BASIC FOOD CHOICES
Meats

You can eat all fresh meats—beef, pork, lamb, buffalo, venison, and game meats. All cuts of meat such as steaks, ribs, roasts, chops, and ground beef, pork, and lamb can be consumed. Red meat from organically raised, grass-fed animals without hormones and antibiotics is preferred. Leave the fat on the meat and eat it. Fat is necessary for proper protein metabolism and enhances the flavor of the meat.

Processed meats that contain nitrates, nitrites, MSG, or sugar should be avoided. This includes most cold cuts and processed meats like hot dogs, bratwurst, sausage, bacon, and ham. However, processed meats with only herbs and spices added are allowed. Read the ingredient labels. If they don't contain chemical additives or sugar they are likely okay to use. If they contain only a small amount of sugar and no other chemicals, you may still use them, as long as you take into account the sugar and add it to your total carbohydrate allotment for the day. If you eat breaded meats or meatloaf you must account for the carbohydrate content.

All forms of fowl are allowed—chicken, turkey, duck, goose, Cornish hen, quail, pheasant, emu, ostrich, and all others. Do not remove the skin; eat it along with the meat. It is often the tastiest part. All eggs are allowed.

All forms of fish and shellfish are allowed—salmon, tuna, sole, trout, catfish, flounder, sardines, herring, crab, lobster, oysters, mussels, clams, and all others. Wild-caught fish is recommended over farm raised. Fish roe or caviar is also allowed.

Most fresh meats do not contain carbohydrate, so you can eat them without doing any calculations on carbohydrate content. The only exceptions are some shellfish and eggs, which do contain a small amount of carbohydrate. A large chicken egg, for instance, contains about a half a gram of carbohydrate.

Processed meats are not free foods. They often have added carbohydrate, so you will need to calculate the carb content using the Nutrition Facts label on the package.

People who go on low-carb diets often miss crispy snacks, such as pretzels, chips, and crackers. These are too high in carbohydrate and often contain unwanted additives such as fructose. A zero-carb alternative is fried pork rinds, sometimes also called pork skins. These are made from the layer of fat under the animal's skin. As the fat is rendered off, only the protein matrix is left. These crispy treats can be eaten as snacks, used in place of croutons in salads, crushed and used as breading in baking fish or chicken, or as a topping on casseroles or other dishes.

Dairy

Some dairy products are relatively high in carbohydrate while others are low. A cup of whole milk contains 11 grams of carbohydrate; 2% has 11.4 grams and 1% has 12.2 grams. As you can see, as the fat content decreases, carbohydrate content increases.

A cup of full-fat plain yogurt contains 12 grams of carbohydrate and a cup of fat-free yogurt contains 19 grams. Sweetened vanilla low-fat yogurt has 31 grams and fruited low-fat yogurt contains about 43 grams.

Most hard cheeses are very low in carbohydrate. Soft cheeses have a little higher carb count but are still not bad. Good cheese choices include cheddar, Colby, Monterey Jack, mozzarella, gruyere, Edam, Swiss, feta, cream cheese (plain), cottage cheese, and goat cheese. An ounce of cheddar cheese has only 0.4 grams of carbs. A full cup of cheddar cheese contains a mere 1.5 grams. A cup of cottage cheese has 8 grams; and a tablespoon of plain cream cheese contains 0.4 grams. Whey cheese and imitation cheese products have a much higher carb content and should be avoided.

Heavy cream has a little over 6 grams of carbs per cup. Half and half contains 10 grams per cup, so you should stick with full-fat cream. A tablespoon of sour cream has 0.5 grams.

You can eat most cheeses and creams without overloading on carbs, but be careful with milk and yogurt. Sweetened dairy products like eggnog, ice cream, and chocolate milk should generally be avoided.

Fats and Oils

Fats and oils contain no carbohydrate, so you can eat as much as you like. Some fats are healthier than others, as you've learned. Choose fats from the "Preferred Fats" category below. All of these oils are safe for food preparation. Steer away from the "Non-Preferred

202

Fats" and never use them in cooking. Completely avoid the "Bad Fats," all foods that contain them, and foods cooked in them such as fries and battered fish.

Preferred Fats	Non-Preferred Fats
Coconut Oil	Corn Oil
Palm Oil/Palm Fruit Oil	Safflower Oil
Palm Shortening	Sunflower Oil
Red Palm Oil	Soybean Oil
Palm Kernel Oil	Cottonseed Oil
Extra Light Olive Oil	Canola Oil
Extra Virgin Olive Oil	Peanut Oil
Macadamia Nut Oil	Walnut Oil
Avocado Oil	Pumpkin Seed Oil
Animal Fat (lard, tallow, meat drippings)	Grapeseed Oil
Butter	**Bad Fats**
Ghee	Margarine
MCT Oil	Shortening
	Hydrogenated Vegetable Oils

Vegetables

You are encouraged to eat plenty of vegetables. Most vegetables are relatively low in carbohydrate. You can easily get the government's recommended five servings per day without going over 25 grams. Serving sizes are generally about ½ cup. A half cup each of cooked cabbage, asparagus, broccoli, mushrooms, and green beans together provides less than 9 grams of carbs. You should eat at least twice this amount every day, along with other appropriate low-carb foods.

Salad greens provide the greatest bulk with the least amount of carbs. Lettuce has less than 1 gram of carbohydrate per cup. A tossed salad consisting of 2 cups of lettuce, 1 cup of mixed low-carb vegetables, and ½ cup of medium-carb vegetables, plus 1 or 2 tablespoons of Italian dressing could easily come to under 9 grams of carbs. You can add cheese and meat without seriously affecting the total carb count. At least one raw salad daily is highly recommended.

Although you are encouraged to eat both raw and cooked vegetables, raw are preferred. When vegetables are cooked, starches and cellulose (fiber) are broken down somewhat and are more easily converted into sugar. For this reason, cooked vegetables tend to raise blood sugar levels more than raw vegetables.

Vegetables are listed below according to their relative carbohydrate content. Vegetables with 6 grams of carbohydrate or less per cup are listed in the low-carb group. Some of these vegetables, particularly leafy greens, have much less than 6 grams. The average carbohydrate content for the vegetables in the low-carb list is about 3 grams per cup. Most of the vegetables you eat should come from this group.

The medium-carb vegetable group has between 7 and 14 grams of carbohydrate per cup. These vegetables should be eaten in moderation. Eating too many can easily send you over the 25 Gram Diet limit and possibly even the 50 Gram Diet limit. A cup of chopped onions contains 14 grams of carbohydrate. However, it isn't often you would want to eat this much onion. A couple of tablespoons or less is more likely. A tablespoon of chopped onion has less than 1 gram of carbs.

High-carb starchy vegetables, like potatoes, are packed with carbohydrate. While no vegetable is strictly off limits, it makes sense for you to avoid high-carb vegetables as a general rule, especially if you are on the 25 Gram Diet. One serving can eat up an entire day's worth of carbohydrate. Even in the 50 gram diet, eating a single serving would severely limit your food choices for the rest of the day. The Low-Carb Prevention Diet may include some starchy vegetables, but these should still be limited to just one meal at the most, and only one serving.

Most types of winter squash are high in carbohydrate. Two exceptions are pumpkin and spaghetti squash, which have about half the carbohydrate as other squashes. Spaghetti squash gets its name from the fact that when it is cooked, it separates into strings resembling spaghetti noodles. These "noodles" can be used as a replacement for pasta. For example, a low-carb spaghetti dish can be made by topping the spaghetti squash with meat and sauce.

Fresh corn is listed in the high-carb category. Technically, corn is a grain and not a vegetable, but it is typically eaten like a vegetable. Corn contains over 25 grams of carbohydrate per cup.

Low-Carb Vegetables
(less than 7g/cup)
Artichoke
Avocado
Asparagus
Bamboo Shoots
Bean Sprouts (mung bean)
Beet Greens
Bok Choy
Broccoli
Brussels Sprouts
Cabbage
Cauliflower
Celery
Celery Root/Celeriac
Chard
Chives
Collard Greens
Cucumber
Daikon Radish
Eggplant
Endive
Fennel
Herbs and Spices
Jicama
Kale
Lettuce (all types)
Mushrooms
Mustard Greens
Napa Cabbage
Okra
Peppers (hot and sweet)
Radish
Rhubarb
Sauerkraut
Scallions
Seaweed (nori, kombu, and
wakame)
Sprouts

Sorrel
Spinach
Snow Peas
String Beans
Summer Squash
Taro Leaves
Tomatillos
Tomato
Turnips
Water Chestnuts
Watercress
Zucchini

Medium-Carb Vegetables
(between 7-14 g/cup)
Beets
Carrot
Kohlrabi
Leeks
Onion
Parsnip
Peas
Rutabaga
Soybean (edamame)
Spaghetti Squash

High-Carb Starchy Vegetables
(over 15 g/cup)
Chickpeas (garbanzo)
Corn (fresh)
Dry Beans (pinto, kidney, etc.)
Jerusalem Artichoke
Lima Beans
Lentils
Potato
Sweet Potato
Taro Root
Winter Squash
Yams

Fruits

A few fruits can be incorporated into the diet if eaten sparingly. Berries have the lowest carbohydrate content of all the fruits. Blackberries and raspberries contain about 7 grams per cup. Strawberries, boysenberries, and gooseberries have a little more, about 9 grams per cup. Blueberries, however, have a much higher carb content, nearly 18 grams per cup. Lemons and limes are also low in carbs, containing less than 4 grams per fruit. Most other fruits typically deliver about 15 to 30 grams of carbohydrate per cup.

With careful planning you can incorporate some low-carb fruits into even the 25 Gram Diet. More fruit can be added to the 50 Gram and Prevention Diets. Because of their high sugar content, fruits should always be eaten in moderation. Choose fresh fruits over canned or frozen, so you will know exactly what you are getting; canned and frozen fruits often have added sugar or syrup.

Dried fruit is extraordinarily sweet because the sugar is concentrated. For example, a cup of fresh grapes contains about 26 grams of carbohydrate while a cup of dried grapes (raisins) contains 109 grams. Dates, figs, currants, raisins, and fruit leathers are so sweet that they are little more than candy.

Low-Carb Fruits	High-Carb Fruits	
Boysenberries	Apple	Melons
Blackberries	Apricot	Mulberries
Gooseberries	Banana	Nectarine
Lemon	Blueberries	Orange
Lime	Cherries	Papaya
Cranberries	Currants	Passion fruit
(unsweetened)	Dates	Peach
Raspberries	Elderberries	Pear
Strawberries	Figs	Persimmon
	Grapefruit	Pineapple
	Grapes	Plum
	Guava	Prunes
	Kiwi	Raisins
	Kumquat	Tangerine
	Mango	

Nuts and Seeds

At first, you might think of nuts and seeds as being high in carbohydrate, but surprisingly, they are only a modest source. For example, 1 cup of sliced almonds contains about 9 grams of carbohydrate. A single whole almond supplies about 0.10 gram.

Most tree nuts deliver about 6 to 10 grams of carbs per cup. Cashews and pistachios pack a higher carbohydrate punch of 40 and 21 grams per cup respectively.

Seeds are generally more carbohydrate rich than nuts. For instance, sesame seeds and sunflower seeds contain about 16 grams per cup.

Black walnuts, pecans, almonds, and coconuts have the lowest carbohydrate content of all the common nuts and seeds. One cup of shredded raw coconut has less than 3 grams of carbohydrate. One cup of dried, desiccated, unsweetened coconut has 7 grams. Canned coconut milk has about 7 grams per cup. In comparison, whole dairy milk with 11 grams per cup. Coconut milk can be a suitable lower carb substitute for dairy milk in most recipes.

All nuts and seeds can be used as toppings on vegetables and salads if the serving size is limited to a tablespoon or two. When eaten as a snack, it is best to stick with the low-carb nuts. The nuts in the low-carb category below contain less than 10 grams of carbohydrate per cup. Those in the high-carb list have 11 grams or more per cup.

Low-Carb Nuts and Seeds	High-Carb Nuts and Seeds
Almond	Cashew
Black Walnut	Peanut
Brazil Nuts	Pine Nuts
Coconut	Pistachio
English Walnut	Pumpkin Seed
Hazelnut (Filbert)	Sesame Seed
Macadamia	Soy Nuts
Pecan	Sunflower Seed

Breads and Grains

Breads and grains are among the highest sources of carbohydrate. On the 25 and 50 Gram Diets you generally need to eliminate all breads, grains, and cereals. This includes wheat, barley, cornmeal, oats, rice, amaranth, arrowroot, millet, quinoa, pasta, couscous, cornstarch, and bran. A single serving can eat up all or most of the day's carbohydrate allotment. A large soft pretzel, for instance, contains 97 grams of carbohydrate; a cup of Froot Loops breakfast cereal supplies 25 grams, and a cup of Raisin Bran cereal contains 39 grams. A cup of Cream of Wheat with a half cup of milk and a spoonful of honey comes to 48 grams of carbohydrate.

Whole grain breads and cereals are generally more nutritious and have a much higher fiber content than refined breads; however, the carbohydrate content is almost the same. A slice of whole wheat bread delivers about 11 grams of carbohydrate, while a slice of white bread has 12 grams; not a big difference.

A small amount of flour or cornstarch can be used to thicken gravies and sauces. One tablespoon of whole wheat flour contains 4.5 grams of carbohydrate and a tablespoon of cornstarch contains 7 grams. This must be calculated into your daily total carbohydrate allotment, so don't use too much. Cornstarch has greater thickening power than wheat or other flours, so a smaller amount can be used to accomplish the same effect.

A non-carb thickening option is cream cheese, which will impart a mild cheesy flavor to the gravy or sauce. Another non-carb but tasteless thickener is xanthan gum, a soluble vegetable fiber commonly used as a thickening agent in processed foods. A similar product is ThickenThin not/Starch thickener. This product can be used to thicken sauces the way cornstarch and flour does, but it has no net carbs, since it is made from fiber. Both ThickenThin not/Starch and xanthan gum powder are available at health food stores and online.

Beverages

Beverages are among the biggest contributors to diabetes and obesity. Most beverages are loaded with sugar and provide little or no nutrition. Sodas and powdered drinks are no more than liquid candy. Even fruit juices and sports drinks are primarily sugar water. One cup (220 ml) of orange juice contains 25 grams of carbs. Vegetable juices are not much better. Many beverages contain caffeine, which is addicting and encourages the overconsumption of sugary beverages. Many people habitually down five, six, or more cups of coffee or cans of cola a day. Some people don't even drink water, relying solely on beverages of one type or another for their daily fluid needs.

The absolute best beverage for the body is water. When the body is dehydrated and needs fluids, it requires water, not Coke or cappuccino. Water satisfies thirst better than any beverage without the added baggage of sugar, caffeine, or chemicals.

Water is, by far, the best option and I encourage you to make it your first choice. You can spike your water or club soda, which is basically carbonated water without sweetening or flavoring, with a little fresh lemon or lime juice to give it flavor. Another option is unsweetened essence-flavored seltzer water. Unsweetened herbal teas and decaffeinated coffee are essentially carb-free. Stay away from all artificially sweetened, low-calorie soft drinks, as artificial sweeteners carry health risks and keep sugar cravings alive and active.

Dehydration increases blood sugar concentration and exacerbates insulin resistance. Most people are slightly dehydrated most of the time. People often ignore their body's internal signals of thirst until dehydration is well underway. Most people would benefit from taking greater effort to drink approved beverages more often. As a rule of thumb, you should drink at least eight 8-ounce (220 ml) servings of water daily. In the summer or when temperatures are hot, you may need to increase this to 10 to 12 servings a day or more.

Condiments

Condiments include herbs, spices, salt, seasonings, salt substitutes, vinegar, mustard, horseradish, relish, hot sauce, fish sauce, and the like. Most condiments are allowed because they are used in such small quantities that the amount of carbohydrate is insignificant; however, there are a few exceptions. Ketchup, sweet pickle relish, barbeque sauce, and some salad dressings are loaded with sugar. In many cases you can find low-carb versions. You need to read the ingredient and Nutrition Facts labels on all prepared foods.

Most salad dressings are made with polyunsaturated vegetable oils. A better choice is olive oil-based or homemade dressings. Vinegar and olive oil or vinegar and water make excellent dressings. Vinegar is especially good, as it is known to improve insulin sensitivity and to lower blood sugar levels by as much as 30 percent after a high-carb meal.[1] The effects of vinegar have been compared favorably to metformin, a popular medication used for blood sugar control.[2] Incorporating a little vinegar into your diet would be beneficial.

Sugar and Sweets

It is best to avoid all sweeteners and foods that contain them, especially on the 25 and 50 Gram Diets. One of the signs of carbohydrate addiction, and a potential or existing blood sugar problem, is a craving for sweets. So-called natural sweeteners such as honey, molasses, sucanat (dehydrated sugarcane juice), agave syrup, and such are no better than white sugar. All foods containing artificial sweeteners and sugar substitutes should also be avoided.

All sweeteners, even natural ones, feed sugar addiction. When the tongue senses sweetness, it doesn't differentiate from granulated sugar, aspartame, or xyitol, and cravings for sweets are maintained. When you are tempted, your willpower will be tested. Once you break down and eat a forbidden sweet, it will be easier to repeat the action the next time temptation arises and, before you know it, you will find yourself hopelessly trapped in the clutches of carbohydrate addiction.

Once you break your addiction to sugar, sweets lose their control over you and become less appealing. You will be able to take them or leave them. They will no longer control you, but you will control them. You will be in charge, and if you do indulge, you will decide when, where, and how much.

Snacks

Occasionally, you may want a snack between meals, though it is important to realize that if you feel hungry in the middle of the day, you may only be thirsty. Simply drinking a glass of water may be enough to stave off these feelings.

If water isn't satisfying enough, there are some low-carb options. Vegetables such as cucumber, daikon radish, and celery make good snacks. Celery sticks can be filled with peanut butter or cream cheese. One tablespoon of peanut butter has 2 grams of carbs, and a tablespoon of plain cream cheese has only 0.5 grams.

If you crave a crispy snack, zero-carb pork rinds may fit the bill. Another crispy snack is nori, a seaweed that is popular in Japanese cooking and is used to wrap sushi. It is commonly sold dried and roasted in paper-thin sheets. Nori has a mild salty seafood flavor. It can be cut into bite-sized squares and eaten like chips and has essentially zero carbs.

Low-carb nuts such as almonds, pecans, and coconut make good snacks. A quarter cup of these nuts supplies about 2.5 grams of carbohydrate.

Meat, cheese, and eggs are other good snack foods. A 1-ounce slice of cheese has about 0.5 grams of carbs. Eggs have about the same. Meat has none, unless it is processed. Some simple snacks are deviled eggs, string cheese, cucumber boats filled with tuna salad, and sliced cheese and ham rolled together with a little mustard or sour cream or rolled around some fresh sprouts.

Store-bought protein bars are popular with low-carbers, but I don't recommend them. They are nothing more than glorified candy bars, often sweetened with artificial sweeteners or sugar substitutes. They are really just a glorified form of processed junk food.

KETOSIS TEST STRIPS

Once a ketogenic diet is started, it takes a few days for blood ketone levels to build up. While we always have some ketones in our blood, the levels are usually too low to be of any therapeutic value. During starvation, fasting, or carbohydrate restriction, ketone production increases. Once the liver's stores of glucose are depleted, ketone production shifts into high gear. After two or three days you will be able to measure the relative amount of ketones in your blood using a urine ketosis test strip, also known as a lipolysis test strip.

One end of the test strip is dipped into a fresh specimen of urine. The strip changes color depending on the ketone concentration in the urine. With the test strip a person can tell if his or her blood ketone level is "none," "trace," "small," "moderate," or "large." The test is helpful in that it indicates whether or not the dietary changes are producing ketones and to what degree. As you add more carbohydrate into the diet, ketone levels drop. To increase ketosis you can reduce carbohydrate consumption.

Generally, the Low-Carb 25 Gram Diet will produce a measurable reading on the test strips. The Low-Carb 50 Gram Diet may or may not produce a reading, depending on how carb sensitive a person is. The Low-Carb Prevention Diet will generally not register on the test strips. The fact that the test strips may indicate "none" does not mean the blood is devoid of all ketones; rather, it means that the ketone level is too low to be detected using the strips. Ketones will, however, be in the blood at a slightly higher level than normal.

Adding coconut oil to these diets will enhance ketone levels. Coconut oil on its own, regardless of diet, will produce some level of ketosis, depending on the amount consumed. Coconut oil will also elevate each of the Low-Carb Diets to a higher level of ketosis. Even the Low-Carb Prevention Diet, with coconut oil added, can potentially produce a measurable reading.

Heavy water consumption may affect the readings. Although blood ketosis levels may be elevated, drinking a lot of water will dilute the urine; this, in turn, will dilute the reading, so you may be in moderate or high ketosis, even if the test strips indicate only "trace" or "none."

Although not required, these test strips can be helpful in encouraging compliance to the program and maintaining carbohydrate restriction. Ketosis test strips are sold in pharmacies; a popular brand is Ketostix.

SUMMARY

Now you have all the tools you need to preserve your eyesight and improve your eye health. Let's summarize the steps you need to take. First you must determine if you want to follow the Low-Carb Prevention Diet or one of the Low-Carb Treatment diets. This is determined by your fasting blood glucose level. The higher your fasting blood glucose is, the more aggressive your diet needs to be to correct this problem.

Your primary food choices should consist of *fresh* produce, meats, eggs, and dairy. You should avoid, as much as possible, processed foods, especially those that contain food additives like hydrogenated vegetable oils, aspartame, and MSG.

Eat healthy fats like coconut oil and red palm oil, especially coconut oil as it is ketogenic and stimulates the production of BDNF, which are so beneficial to the brain and eyes. Keep in mind that fats improve the absorption of the nutrients in your foods. Your diet should include plenty of fat. Your diet should *not* be low-fat. The Low-Carb Prevention Diet recommends 1 to 3 tablespoons (15 to 45 ml) of added coconut oil and the treatment diets 4 to 5 tablespoons (60 to 74 ml) daily. This is in addition to the fats already present in the foods. You should, however, avoid all refined polyunsaturated vegetable oils and foods that contain them. Get into the habit of reading ingredient labels.

Your diet should contain lots of fresh vegetables, both cooked and raw, which will provide you with an abundant source of eye healthy vitamins, minerals, and antioxidants. This diet should provide you with an ample amount of vitamin A, an essential nutrient for good eye health, from meat, fish, eggs, and dairy as well as provitamin A carotenoids from richly colored vegetables. However, if desired, you can add some dietary supplements. The most important for eye health are lutein, zeaxanthin, and astaxanthin.

Avoid all forms of tobacco and discontinue all unnecessary drugs. Tobacco and drugs are among the most damaging influences to the eyes. Removing them from your life can make a big difference with your eye health. A major benefit with this program it that your need for prescription and over-the-counter medications will diminish. If you follow the program as described, you can eliminate the need for the majority of commonly used medications, including those for high cholesterol, high blood pressure, high blood sugar and diabetes, and many others. Work with your doctor to reduce your prescriptions and ween yourself off of over-the-counter medications.

Overexposure to sunlight can adversely affect eye health, this is particularly true if you have a poor diet. A diet rich in good fats and antioxidant nutrients will protect you from much of the damage UV radiation from the sun can otherwise cause. Once you begin to eat a vegetable-rich, low-carb diet, your resistance to UV radiation will increase dramatically and you will not have to be extraordinarily cautious about avoiding the sun. The sun's rays can actually be healthful and provide the best source of vitamin D—an essential hormone-like vitamin synthesized in the skin by UV light. So, some sun exposure is necessary for good health.

Periodically you should have your fasting blood glucose or A1C levels checked. Over time, your blood sugar levels should improve, even without medication. This is a clear sign your overall health is improving and your risk of visual impairment is decreasing.

As with any treatment or prevention program, the closer you can follow the program as outlined, the better the results. Give it time. You are working on a cellular level here. The nutrients in your diet are protecting and strengthening your eyes little by little, cell by cell. Your eyesight may remain stable, rather than degenerate, or may gradually improve. While you may still experience presbyopia—the normal vision loss due to aging, your resistance to eye diseases—abnormal conditions—such as cataracts, macular degeneration, glaucoma, diabetic retinopathy, dry eye syndrome, and others will be greatly reduced. In many cases, if you follow the stricter Low-Carb Treatment programs you may experience a reversal in symptoms associated with these conditions.

Net Carbohydrate Counter

Food	Amount	Net Carbs (g)
Vegetables		
Alfalfa sprouts	1 cup/33 g	0.5
Artichoke, boiled	1 medium/120 g*	6.5
Arugula	1 cup/20 g	0.5
Asparagus, raw	4 spears/1 cup/60 g	2
Avocado (Haas)	1 each/173 g*	3.5
Bamboo shoots, canned	1 cup/131 g	2.5
Beans, boiled, drained		
black	1 cup/172 g	26
black-eyed peas	1 cup/172 g	15
garbanzo (chickpeas)	1 cup/164 g	34
great northern	1 cup/177 g	26
green beans, fresh	1 cup/100 g	7
kidney	1 cup/170 g	27
lentils	1 cup/198 g	30
lima	1 cup/172 g	24
navy	1 cup/182 g	32
pinto	1 cup/898 g	24
soybeans	1 cup/172 g	12
Bean sprouts (mung)		
boiled	1 cup/124 g	2
raw	1 cup/104 g	3

*The amount indicated is for the edible portion, less skin, core, pit, seeds, etc.

Food	Amount	Net Carbs (g)
Beets (sliced), raw	1 cup/170 g	8
Beet greens, boiled	1 cup/144 g	5
Broccoli, raw, chopped	1 cup/88 g	2
Brussels sprouts, boiled	1 cup/156 g	8
Cabbage, green, shredded		
cooked	1 cup/150 g	3
raw	1 cup/70 g	2
Cabbage, red, shredded		
cooked	1 cup/150 g	3
raw	1 cup/70 g	2
Chinese cabbage		
(bok choy)		
cooked	1 cup/170 g	1
raw	1 cup/170 g	1
Carrot		
boiled, chopped	1 cup/156 g	10
raw, whole	1 medium/72 g	5
raw, shredded	1 cup/110 g	8
juice	1 cup/246 g	18
Cauliflower		
boiled	1 cup/124 g	1.5
raw, chopped	1 cup/100 g	2.5
Celery		
raw, whole	8 in long/40 g	1
raw, diced	1 cup/120 g	2
Chard		
boiled	1 cup/175 g	3.5
raw	1 cup/36 g	1.5
Chives, chopped	1 tbsp/6 g	0
Collards		
boiled, drained	1 cup/190 g	4
raw	1 cup/37 g	0.5
Cucumber, sliced		
raw with peel	1 cup/119 g	3
Daikon, raw	4 in/10 cm long	6

Food	Amount	Net Carbs (g)
Eggplant, raw	1 cup/82 g	2
Escarole, raw	1 cup/50 g	0.5
Garlic, raw	1 clove	1
Jerusalem artichoke, raw	1 cup/150 g	24
Jicama, raw	1 cup/130 g	5
Kale, chopped, boiled	1 cup/130 g	3
Kelp, raw	1 oz/28 g	2
Kohlrabi		
cooked, sliced	1 cup/140 g	7
raw, sliced	1 cup/165 g	9
Leeks, raw	1 cup/104 g	13
Lettuce		
butterhead	2 leaves/15 g	0
iceberg	1 wedge/135 g	1
iceberg, shredded	1 cup/56 g	0.5
loose leaf, chopped	1 cup/56 g	0.5
romaine, chopped	1 cup/56 g	0.5
Mushrooms (button)		
boiled	1 cup/156 g	4
raw, sliced	1 cup/70 g	2.5
raw	3 mushrooms	1
Mustard greens		
raw	1 cup/60 g	1
boiled	1 cup/140 g	0.5
Okra, raw, sliced	1 cup/184 g	12
Onion		
raw, sliced	1 cup/115 g	8
raw, chopped	1 cup/160 g	11
raw, whole medium	2.5 in/6.4 cm dia	10
Parsley		
raw, chopped	1 tbsp/4 g	0
Parsnips		
raw, chopped	1 cup/110 g	17.5
Peas		
edible-pod, cooked	1 cup/160 g	7

Food	Amount	Net Carbs (g)
green, boiled	1 cup/160 g	7
split, boiled	1 cup/196 g	31
Peppers		
hot red chili, raw	½ cup/68 g	3
jalapeno, canned	½ cup/68 g	1
sweet (bell), raw,	1 cup/50 g	2
sweet (bell), raw	1 medium	4
Potatoes		
baked, with skin	1 medium/202 g	46
baked, without skin	1 medium/156 g	32
mashed, with milk	1 cup/210 g	34
hash brown		
cooked in oil	1 cup/156 g	41
Pumpkin, canned	1 cup/245 g	15
Radish, raw	10 radishes/45 g	1
Rhubarb, raw, copped	1 cup/122 g	3.5
Rutabaga, chopped,		
cooked	1 cup/170 g	12
Sauerkraut, canned		
with liquid	1 cup/236 g	6
Scallions		
raw, chopped	½ cup/50 g	3
raw, whole	4 in/10 cm long	1
Shallots, raw, minced	1 tbsp/10 g	1
Spinach		
cooked, drained	1 cup/180 g	3
raw, chopped	1 cup/56 g	1
Sprouts, see Alfalfa		
Squash, winter verities		
crookneck, raw, sliced	1 cup/180 g	5
scallop, raw sliced	1 cup/113 g	3
zucchini, raw sliced	1 cup/180 g	3
Squash, summer varieties		
acorn, baked, mashed	1 cup/245 g	29
butternut, baked,		
mashed	1 cup/245 g	19

Food	Amount	Net Carbs (g)
Hubbard, baked, mashed	1 cup/240 g	20
spaghetti, baked	1 cup/155	6
Sweet potato, baked	1 med,4 oz/114 g	25
Taro		
root, cooked, sliced	1 cup/104 g	24
leaves, raw, chopped	1 cup/28 g	1
Tofu	½ cup/126 g	1
Tomato		
cooked/stewed	1 cup/240 g	10
raw, chopped	1 cup/180 g	5
raw, sliced	0.25 in/0.6 cm thick	1
raw, whole	1 med, 4.3 oz/123 g	4
raw	1 lg, 6.4 oz/181 g	5
cherry	2 med, 1.2 oz/34 g	1
Italian	1 med, 2.2 oz/62 g	2
juice	1 cup/244 g	8
paste	½ cup/131 g	19
sauce	½ cup/122 g	7
Turnips, raw	1 med	6
Turnip greens, raw	1 cup/55g	1.5
Water chestnuts, sliced	½ cup/70 g	7
Watercress, raw chopped	½ cup/17 g	0
Yam, baked	1 cup/150 g	36

Fruit _____

Apples		
raw	1 each/138 g*	18
juice	1 cup/248 g	29
applesauce, unsweetened	1 cup/244 g	24
Apricots		
raw	1 each	3
canned, in syrup	1 cup/258 g	51
Banana	1 each/114 g*	25

*The amount indicated is for the edible portion, less skin, core, pit, seeds, etc.

Food	Amount	Net Carbs (g)
Blackberries, fresh	1 cup/144 g	8
Blueberries, fresh	1 cup/145 g	17
Boysenberries, frozen	1 cup/132 g	9
Cantaloupe	½ each/267 g	19
Cherries, sweet, raw	10 each/68 g	9.5
Cranberry		
Raw	1 cup/95 g	7
Sauce, whole berry		
canned	1 cup/277 g	102
Dates, raw		
whole without pits	10 each/83 g	54
chopped	1 cup/178 g	116
Elderberries, raw	1 cup/145 g	16.5
Figs	10 each/187 g	101
Gooseberries, raw	1 cup/150 g	9
Grapefruit, raw	1 half/91 g	7
Grapes		
Thompson seedless	10 each/50 g	8
American (slip skin)	10 each/50 g	4
juice, canned	1 cup/236 ml	37
juice, from		
frozen concentrate	1 cup/236 ml	31
Honeydew	1 cup/6 oz/170 g*	14
Kiwi, raw	1 each/76 g*	8
Lemon, raw	1 each	4
Lemon Juice	1 tbsp/15 ml	1
Lime, raw	1 each	3
Lime Juice	1 tbsp/15 ml	1
Loganberries, frozen	1 cup/147 g	11
Mandarin orange		
canned, juice pack	1 cup/250 g	22
canned, light syrup	1 cup/250 g	39
Mango, raw	1 each/207 g*	28
Mulberries, raw	1 cup/138 g	11
Nectarines, raw	1 each/136 g*	13

Food	Amount	Net Carbs (g)
Olives		
black	10 each	2
green	10 each	1
Oranges, raw	1 each/248 g*	12
Juice, fresh	1 cup/236 ml	25
Juice, from		
frozen concentrate	1 cup/236 ml	27
Papayas, raw, sliced	1 cup/140 g*	12
Peaches		
raw, whole	1 each/87 g*	8
raw sliced	1 cup/153 g	14
canned, heavy syrup	1 cup/256 g	48
canned, juice packed	1 cup/248 g	26
Pears		
raw	1 each/166 g*	20
canned, heavy syrup	1 cup/255 g	45
canned, juice packed	1 cup/248 g	28
Persimmon, raw	1 each	8.5
Pineapple,		
fresh, cubed	1 cup/155 g	17
crushed/cubed, packed		
in heavy syrup	1 cup/255 g	50
crushed/cubed,		
juice packed	1 cup/250 g	37
Plantains, cooked, sliced	1 cup/154 g*	41
Plums, raw	1 each/66 g*	7.5
Prunes		
dried	10 each/84 g	45
juice	1 cup/236 ml	42
Raisins	1 cup/145 g	106
Raspberries, raw	1 cup/123 g	6
Strawberries		
raw, whole	1 each	1
raw, halves	1 cup/153 g	8
raw, sliced	1 cup/167 g	9

Food	Amount	Net Carbs (g)
Tangerines, fresh	1 each/84 g*	7.5
Watermelon		
sliced	1 inch/2.5 cm	33
balls	1 cup/160 g	11

Nuts and Seeds

Food	Amount	Net Carbs (g)
Almonds		
sliced or slivered	1 cup/95 g	9
whole	1 oz/28 g	3
almond butter	1 tbsp/16 g	2
Brazil nuts	1 oz/28 g	1.5
Cashew		
halves and whole	1 cup/137 g	37
whole	1 oz/28 g	6
cashew butter	1 tbsp/16 g	3
Coconut		
fresh	2 x 2 in/5 x 5 cm	2
fresh, shredded	1 cup/80 g	3
dried, unsweetened	1 cup/78 g	7
dried, sweetened	1 cup/93 g	35
Filberts (hazelnuts)		
whole	1 oz/28 g	2
whole	1 cup/118 g	11
Macadamia		
whole	1 oz/28 g	1.5
whole or halves	1 cup/134 g	7
Peanuts		
oil roasted	1 cup/144 g	14
oil roasted	1 oz/28 g	3
peanut butter	1 tbsp/16 g	2
Pecans		
halves, raw	1 cup/108 g	5
halves, raw	1 oz/28 g	3
Pine nuts		
whole	1 oz/28 g	3

Food	Amount	Net Carbs (g)
Pistachio		
Whole, roasted	1 oz/28 g	6
Whole, roasted	1 cup/128 g	21
Pumpkin seeds		
whole	1 oz/28 g	3
whole	1 cup/227 g	11
Sesame seeds		
whole	1 tbsp/9.5 g	1
sesame butter (tahini)	1 tbsp/15 g	2
Soy nuts, roasted	1 oz/28 g	5
Sunflower seeds		
whole, hulled	1 tbsp/8.5 g	1
Walnuts		
Black	1 oz/28 g	1
black, chopped	1 cup/125 g	4
English	1oz/28 g	3
English, chopped	1 cup/120 g	8

Grains and Flours

Amaranth, whole grain	1 cup/192 g	100
Arrowroot flour	1 tbsp/8.5 g	7
Barley		
pearled, uncooked	1 cup/200 g	127
pearled, cooked	1 cup/157 g	40
flour	1 cup/124 g	95
Buckwheat		
whole grain	1 cup/175 g	112
flour	1 cup/98 g	73
Bulgur		
whole grain, cooked	1 cup/182 g	23
flour	1 cup/140 g	75
Coconut flour	1 cup/114 g	24
Corn		
whole kernel	1 cup/210 g	38
ear, small	6 in/15 cm long	12

Food	Amount	Net Carbs (g)
ear, medium	7 in/18 cm long	15
ear, large	8.5 in/22 cm long	23
grits, uncooked	1 cup/156 g	122
grits, cooked with water	1 cup/240 g	30
cornmeal, dry	1 cup/122 g	81
corn starch	1 tbsp/8.5 g	7
popcorn, air popped	1 cup/8.5 g	5
hominy, canned	1 cup/260 g	20
Millet		
uncooked	1 cup/200 g	129
cooked	1 cup/240 g	54
Oats		
oatmeal, cooked	1 cup/234 g	21
oatmeal, uncooked	1 cup/100 g	46
oat bran, uncooked	¼ cup/25 g	13
Quinoa		
uncooked	1 cup/170 g	98
cooked	1 cup/184 g	34
Rice		
brown, cooked	1 cup/195 g	42
white, cooked	1 cup/205 g	56
instant, cooked	1 cup/165 g	34
wild rice, cooked	1 cup/164 g	32
brown rice flour	1 cup/159 g	114
white rice flour	1 cup/159 g	123
Rye flour	1 cup/102	64
Semolina flour, enriched	1 cup/167 g	115
Soy flour	1 cup/88 g	24
Tapioca		
pearl dry	1 cup/152 g	133
flour	1 tbsp/8 g	7
Wheat		
white, flour	1 cup/128 g	92
white, flour	1 tbsp/8 g	6

Food	Amount	Net Carbs (g)
whole wheat flour	1 cup/120 g	72
whole wheat flour	1 tbsp/7.5 g	5
wheat bran	½ cup/30 g	11

Bread and Baked Goods

Bagels
white enriched	1 ea (3.7 oz/105 g)	57
whole grain	1 ea (4.5 oz/128 g)	64

Bread
rye	1 slice	13
whole wheat	1 slice	11
white	1 slice	12
raisin bread	1 slice	13
hamburger bun	1 roll	20
hot dog bun	1 roll	20
hard/Kaiser roll	1 roll	29

Crackers
Saltine	1 each	2
wheat	1 each	1
cheese	1 each	1
English muffin	1 each	24
Pancake	1 ea (4 in/10 cm dia)	13

Pita
white	1 each	32
whole wheat	1 each	31

Tortilla
corn	1 ea (6 in/15 cm)	11
flour	1 ea (8 in/20 cm)	22
flour	1 ea (10.5 in/27 cm)	34
Wonton wrappers	1 ea (3.5 in/9 cm)	5

Pasta

Macaroni, cooked
white, enriched	1 cup/140 g	38
whole wheat	1 cup/140 g	35

Food	Amount	Net Carbs (g)
corn	1 cup/140 g	32
Noodles, cooked		
cellophane		
(mung bean)	1 cup/190 g	39
egg	1 cup/160 g	36
soba	1 cup/113 g	19
rice	1 cup/175 g	42
Spaghetti, cooked		
white, enriched	1 cup/140 g	38
whole wheat	1 cup/140 g	32
corn	1 cup/140 g	32

Dairy

Food	Amount	Net Carbs (g)
Almond milk	1 cup/236 ml	7
Butter	1 tbsp/14 g	0
Buttermilk	1 cup/236 ml	12
Cheese (hard)		
American, sliced	1 oz/28 g	0.5
Cheddar, sliced	1 oz/28 g	0.5
Cheddar, shredded	1 cup/113 g	1.5
Colby, sliced	1 oz/28 g	0.5
Colby, shredded	1 cup/113 g	3
Edam, sliced	1 oz/28 g	0.5
Edam, shredded	1 cup/113 g	1.5
Gruyere, sliced	1 oz/28 g	0
Gruyere, shredded	1 cup/113 g	0.5
Monterey, sliced	1 oz/28 g	0
Monterey, shredded	1 cup/113 g	1
mozzarella, sliced	1 oz/28 g	0.5
mozzarella, shredded	1 cup/113 g	2.5
Muenster, sliced	1 oz/28 g	0
Muenster, shredded	1 cup/113 g	1
Parmesan, sliced	1 oz/28 g	1
Parmesan, grated	1 tbsp/5 g	0
Swiss, sliced	1 oz/28 g	1.5

Food	Amount	Net Carbs (g)
Swiss, shredded	1 cup/113 g	6
Cheese (soft)		
Brie	1 oz/28 g	1
Camembert	1 oz/28 g	0
cottage, non-fat	1 cup/226 g	9.5
cottage, 2% fat	1 cup/226 g	8
cream cheese, plain	1 tbsp/14 g	0.5
cream cheese, low-fat	1 tbsp/14 g	1
feta, crumbled	1 oz/28 g	1
ricotta, whole milk	1 oz/28 g	1
ricotta, whole milk	1 cup/246 g	7.5
ricotta, part skim	1 oz/28 g	1.5
ricotta, part skim	1 cup/246 g	12.5
Coconut milk, canned	1 cup/236 ml	7
Coconut milk beverage,		
carton	1 cup/236 ml	7
Cream		
heavy whipping	1 cup/236 ml	6.5
half and half	1 cup/236 ml	10.5
sour	1 tbsp/28 g	0.5
Goat milk	1 cup/236 ml	11
Milk		
skim, non-fat	1 cup/236 ml	12
1%	1 cup/236 ml	12
2%	1 cup/236 ml	11.5
whole, 3.3% fat	1 cup/236 ml	11
Kefir	1 cup/236 ml	9
Rice milk		
plain	1 cup/236 ml	23
vanilla	1 cup/236 ml	26
Soy milk	1 cup/236 ml	7
Yogurt		
plain, fat-free	1 cup/227 g	19
plain, low-fat	1 cup/227 g	16
plain, whole milk	1 cup/227 g	12

Food	Amount	Net Carbs (g)
vanilla, low-fat	1 cup/227 g	31
fruit added, low-fat	1 cup/227 g	43

Meat and Eggs

Food	Amount	Net Carbs (g)
Beef	3 oz/85 g	0
Eggs	1 large	0.5
Egg yolk	1 large	0.5
Egg white	1 large	0
Fish		
bass	3 oz/85 g	0
cod	3 oz/85 g	0
flounder	3 oz/85 g	0
haddock	3 oz/85 g	0
Pollock	3 oz/85 g	0
salmon	3 oz/85 g	0
sardines, canned, drained	3 oz/85 g	0
trout	3 oz/85 g	0
tuna, canned, water packed	3 oz/85 g	0
Lamb chop	3 oz/85 g	0
Poultry		
chicken, dark meat	1 cup/140 g	0
chicken, dark meat	3 oz/85 g	0
chicken, light meat	1 cup/140 g	0
chicken, light meat	3 oz/85 g	0
duck	½ duck/221 g	0
turkey, dark meat	3 oz/85 g	0
turkey, light meat	3 oz/85 g	0
turkey, ground	3 oz/85 g	0
Pork		
bacon, cured	3 pieces	0.5
Canadian-style bacon	2 pieces	1
chops	3 oz/85 g	0
fresh side (uncured bacon)	3 oz/85 g	0

Food	Amount	Net Carbs (g)
ham	3 oz/85 g	1
Sausage		
frankfurter, beef/pork	1 ea/57 g	1
frankfurter, chicken	1 ea/45 g	3
frankfurter, turkey	1 ea/45 g	1
bratwurst	1 ea/70 g	2
kielbasa	1 ea/26 g	1
Polish	1 ea/28 g	0
pork, link (large)	1 ea/68 g	1
pork, link (small)	1 ea/13 g	0
salami, beef/pork	2 pices/57 g	1
Shellfish		
clams, canned	3 oz/85 g	4
crab, cooked	1 cup/135 g	0
lobster, cooked	1 cup/145 g	2
mussels, cooked	1 oz/28 g	2
oysters, raw	1 cup/248 g	10
scallops	3 oz/85 g	1
shrimp, cooked	3 oz/85 g	0
Venison	3 oz/85 g	0

Miscellaneous

Baking soda	1 tsp/9 g	0
Catsup		
regular	1 tbsp/15 g	4
low-carb	1 tbsp/15 g	1
Fats and oils	1 tbsp/14 g	0
Gelatin, dry	1 envelope/7 g	0
Fish sauce	1 tbsp/15 ml	0.5
Herbs and spices	1 tbsp/5 g	2
Honey	1 tbsp/21 g	17
Horseradish, prepared	1 tbsp/15 g	1.5
Maple syrup	1 tbsp/15 ml	13.5
Mayonnaise	1 tbsp/14 g	0
Molasses	1 tbsp/20 g	15

Food	Amount	Net Carbs (g)
Molasses, blackstrap	1 tbsp/20 g	12
Mustard		
yellow	1 tbsp/15 g	0
Dijon	1 tbsp/15 g	0
Pancake syrup	1 tbsp/15 g	15
Pickles		
dill, medium	1 pickle/65 g	3
dill, slice	1 (0.2 oz/6 g)	1
sweet, medium	1 pickle/35 g	11
pickle relish, sweet	1 tbsp/15 g	5
Tartar sauce	1 tbsp/15 g	2
Salsa	1 tbsp/15 g	1
Soy sauce	1 tbsp/15 ml	1
Sugar		
white, granulated	1 tbsp/11 g	12
brown, unpacked	1 tbsp/8 g	9
powdered	1 tbsp/8 g	8
Vinegar		
apple cider	1 tbsp/15 ml	0
balsamic	1 tbsp/15 ml	2
red wine	1 tbsp/15 ml	0
rice	1 tbsp/15 ml	0
Worcestershire sauce	1 tbsp/15 ml	3

References

Chapter 2: The Human Eye
1. http://www.who.int/mediacentre/factsheets/fs282/en/

Chapter 3: Common Eye Disorders
1. Babizhayev, MA, et al. Lipid peroxidation and cataracts: N-acetylcarnosine as a therapeutic tool to manage age-related cataracts in human and in canine eyes. *Drugs R D* 2004;5:125-139.
2. Spencer RW and Andelman SY. Steroid cataracts. Posterior subcapsular cataract formation in rheumatoid arthritis patients on long term steroid therapy. *Arch Ophthalmol* 1965;74:38–41.
3. Bonnefont-Rousselot D. Antioxidant and anti-AGE therapeutics. *J Soc Biol* 2001;195: 391–398.
4. Babizhayev, MA, et al. N-acetylcarnosine lubricant eyedrops possess all-in-one universal antioxidant protective effects of L-carnosine in aqueous and lipid membrane environments, aldehyde scavenging, and traansglycation activities inherent to cataracts: a clinical study of the new vision-saving drug N-acetylcarnosine eyedrop therapy in a database population of over 50,500 patients. *Am J Ther* 2009;16:517-533.

Chapter 4: Vision Busters
1. Kowluru, RA and Chan, PS. Oxidative stress and diabetic retinopathy. *Exp Diabetes Res* 2007;2007:43603.
2. Chiu, CJ and Taylor, A. Nutritional antioxidants and age-related cataract and maculopathy. *Exp Eye Res* 2007;84:229-245.
3. Babizhayev, MA and Costa, EB. Lipid peroxide and reactive oxygen species generating systems of the crystalline lens. *Biochim Biophys Acta* 1994;1225:326-337.

4. Babizhayev, MA. Biomarkers and special features of oxidative stress in the anterior segment of the eye linked to lens cataract and the trabecular meshwork injury in primary open-angle glaucoma. *Fundam Clin Pharmacol* 2012;26:86-117.

5. Milne, R and Brownstein, S. Advanced glycation end products and diabetic retinopathy. *Amino Acids* 2013;44:1397-1407.

6. Ishibashi, T, et al. Advanced glycation end products in age-related macular degeneration. *Arch Ophthalmol* 1998;116:1629-1632.

7. Gul, A, et al. Advanced glycation end products in senile diabetic and nondiabetic patients with cataract. *J Diabetes Complications* 2009;23:343-348.

8. Sasaki, N, et al. Advanced glycation end products in Alzheimer's disease and other neurodegenerative diseases. *American Journal of Pathology* 1998;153:1149-1155.

9. Catellani, R, et al. Glycooxidation and oxidative stress in Parkinson's disease and diffuse Lewy body disease. *Brain Res* 1996;737:195-200.

10. Kato, S, et al. Astrocytic hyaline inclusions contain advanced glycation endproducts in familial amyotrophic lateral sclerosis with superoxide dismutase 1 gene mutation: immunohistochemical and immunoelectron microscopical analysis. *Aca Neuropathol* 1999;97:260-266.

11. Krajcovicová-Kudlacková, M, et al. Advanced glycation end products and nutrition. *Physiol Res* 2002;51:313-316.

12. Das, BN, et al. The prevalence of age related cataract in the Asian community in Leicester: a community based study. *Eye (Lond)* 1990;4(Pt 5):723-726.

13. Glenn, JV and Stitt, AW. The role of advanced glycation end products in retinal ageing and disease. *Biochim Biophys Acta* 2009;1790:1109-1116.

14. Milne, R and Brownstein, S. Advanced glycation end products and diabetic retinopathy. *Amino Acids* 2013;44:1397-1407.

15. Taylor, HR, et al. The long-term effects of visible light on the eye. *Arch Ophthalmol* 1992;110:99-104.

16. Cruickshanks, KJ, et al. Sunlight and age-related macular degeneration. The Beaver Dam Eye Study. *Arch Ophthalmol* 1993;111:514-518.

17. van den Berg, TJ, et al. Dependence of intraocular straylight on pigmentation and light transmission through the ocular wall. *Vision Res* 1991;31:1361-1367.

18. Armstrong, D and Hiramitsu, T. Studies of experimentally induced retinal degeneration: 2 Early morphological changes produced by lipid peroxides in the albino rabbit. *Jpn J Ophthalmol* 1990;34:158-173.

19. Cerami, C, et al. Tobacco smoke is a source of toxic reactive glycation products. *Proc Natl Acad Sci USA* 1997;94:13915-13920.

20. Boustani, M, et al. The association between cognition and histamine-2 receptor antagonists in African Americans. *J Am Geriatr Soc* 2007;55:1248-1253.

21. Fliesler, S and Bretillon, L. The ins and outs of cholesterol in the vertebrate retina. *J Lipid Res* 2010;51:3399-3413.

22. Vorwerk, CK, et al. An experimental basis for implicating excitotoxicity in glaucomatous optic neuropathy. *Surv Ophthalmol* 1999;43 Suppl1:S142-S150.

23. Casson, RJ. Possible role of excitotoxicity in the pathogenesis kof glaucoma. *Clin Experiment Ophthalmol* 2006;34:54-63.

24. Choi, D. Glutamate neurotoxicity and diseases of the nervous system. *Neuron* 1988;1:623-34.

25. Lipton, S and Rosenberg, P. Excitatory amino acids as a final common pathway for neurologic disorders. *N Engl J Med* 1994;330:613-22.

26. Whetsell, W and Shapira, N. Biology of disease. Neuroexcitation, excitotoxicity and human neurological disease. *Lab Invest* 1993;68:372-387.

27. Olney, J., et al. Excitotoxic neurodegeneration in Alzheimer's disease. *Arch Neurol* 1997;54:1234-1240.

28. Hynd, MR, et al. Glutamate-mediated excitotoxicity and neurodegeneration in Alzheimer's disease. *Neurochem Int* 2004;45:583-595.

29. Caudle, WM and Zhang, J. Glutamate, excitotoxicity, and programmed cell death in Parkinson disease. *Exp Neurol* 2009;220:230-233.

30. Foran, E and Trotti, D. Glutamate transporters and the excitotoxic path to motor neuron degeneration in amyotrophic lateral sclerosis. *Antioxid Redox Signal* 2009;11:1587-1602.

31. Kort, JJ. Impairment of excitatory amino acid transport in astroglial cells infected with human immunodeficiency virus type I AIDS. *Res Human Retroviruses* 1998;14:1329-1339.

32. Tritti, D and Danbolt, NC. Glutamate transporters are oxidant-vulnerable: a molecular link between oxidative and excitotoxic neurodegeneration. *TIPS* 1998;19:328-334.

33. Blanc, EM, et al. 4-hydroxynonenal, a lipid peroxidation product, impairs glutamate transport in cortical astrocytes. *Glia* 1998;22:149-160.

34. Koenig, H, et al. Capillary NMDA receptors regulate blood-brain barrier function and breakdown. *Bran Res* 1992;588:297-303.

35. Van Westerlaak, MG, et al. Chronic mitochondrial inhibition induces glutamate-mediated corticomotoneuron death in an organotypic culture model. *Exp Neurol* 2001;167:393-400.

Chapter 5: Blood Sugar and Insulin Resistance

1. de la Monte, SM, et al. Impaired insulin and insulin-like growth factor

expression and signaling mechanisms in Alzheimer's disease—is this type 3 diabetes? *J Alzheimers Dis* 2005;7:63-80.

2. Whitmer, RA Type 2 diabetes and risk of cognitive impairment and dementia. *Curr Neurol Neurosci Rep* 2007;7:3730380.

3. Ott, A, et al. Diabetes and the risk of dementia: Rotterdam study. *Neurology* 1999;53:1937-1942.

4. Xu, W, et al. Mid- and late-life diabetes in relation to the risk of dementia: a population-based twin study. *Diabetes* 2009;58:71-77.

5. Ristow, M. Neurodegenerative disorders associated with diabetes mellitus. *J Mol Med* 2004;82:510-529.

6. Craft, S and Watson, GS. Insulin and neurodegenerative disease: shared and specific mechanisms. *Lancet Neurol* 2004;3:169-178.

7. Pradat, PF, et al. Impaired glucose tolerance in patients with amyotrophic lateral sclerosis. *Amyotroph Lateral Scler* 2010;11:166-171.

8. Morris, JK, et al. Measures of striatal insulin resistance in a 6-hydroxydopamine model of Parkinson's disease. *Brain Res* 2008;1240:185-195.

9. Moroo, I, et al. Loss of insulin receptor immunoreactivity from the substantia nigra pars compacta neurons in Parkinson's disease. *Acta Neuropathol* 1994;87:343-348.

10. Sandyk, R. The relationship between diabetes mellitus and Parkinson's disease. *Int J Neurosci* 1993;69:125-130.

11. Hu, G, et al. Type 2 diabetes and the risk of Parkinson's disease. *Diabetes Care* 2007;30:842-847.

12. Oh, SW, et al. Elevated intraocular pressure is associated with insulin resistance and metabolic syndrome. *Diabetes Metab Res Rev* 2005;21:434-440.

13. Pasquale, LR, et al. Prospective study of type 2 diabetes mellitus and risk of primary open-angle glaucoma in woman. *Ophthalmology* 2006;113:1081-1086.

14. Voutilainen-Kaunisto, RM, et al. Age-related macular degeneration in newly diagnosed type 2 diabetic patients and control subjects: a 10-year follow-up on evolution, risk factors, and prognostic significance. *Diabetes Care* 2000;23:672-678.

15. Whitney, EN, et al. *Understanding Normal and Clinical Nutrition*, Third Edition. West Publishing Company, St. Paul, MN, 1991.

16. Rodriguez, RR and Krehal, WA. The influence of diet and insulin on the incidence of cataracts in diabetic rats. *Yale J Biol Med* 1951;24:103-108.

17. The effect of intensive treatment of diabetes on the development and progression of long-term complications in insulin-dependent diabetes mellitus. The Diabetes Control and Complications Research Group. *N Engl J Med* 1993;329:977-986.

18. Chiu, CJ, et al. Carbohydrate intake and glycemic index in relation to the odds of early cortical and nuclear lens opacities. *Am J Clin Nutr* 2005;81:1411-1416.

19. Stratton, IM, et al. Association of glycaemia with macrovascular and microvascular complications of type 2 diabetes (UKPDS 35): prospective observational study. *BMJ* 2000;321:405-412.

20. The effect of intensive diabetes treatment on the progression of diabetic retinopathy in insulin-dependent diabetes mellitus. The Diabetes Control and Complications Trial. *Arch Ophthalmol* 1995;113:36-51.

21. Kerti, L, et al. Higher glucose levels associated with lower memory and reduced hippocampal microstructure. *Neurology* 2013;81:1745-1752.

22. Warram, JH, et al. Slow glucose removal rate and hyperinsulinemia precede the development of type 2 diabetes in the offspring of diabetic parents. *Ann Intern Med* 1990;113:909-915.

Chapter 6: What You Should Know About Fats and Oils

1. Davis, GP and Park, E. *The Heart: The Living Pump*. Torstar Books, New York, 1983.

2. Aruoma, OI and Halliwell, B. eds. *Free Radicals and Food Additives*. Taylor and Francis, London, 1991.

3. Harman, D, et al. Free radical theory of aging: effect of dietary fat on central nervous system function. *J Am Geriatr Soc* 1976;24:301-307.

4. Anderson, RE, et al. Lipid peroxidation and retinal degeneration. *Current Eye Research* 1984;3:223-227.

5. Armstrong, D, et al. Studies on experimentally induced retinal degeneration. 1. Effect of lipid peroxides on electroretinographic activity in the albino rabbit. *Exp Eye Res* 1982;35:157-171.

6. Armstrong, D and Hiramitsu, T. Studies of experimentally induced retinal degeneration: 2 Early morphological changes produced by lipid peroxides in the albino rabbit. *Jpn J Ophthalmol* 1990;34:158-173.

7. Catala, A. An overview of lipid peroxidation with emphasis in outer segments of photoreceptors and the chemiluminescence assay. *Int J Biochem Cell Biol* 2006;38:1482-1495.

8. Seddon, JM, et al. Dietary fat and risk for advanced age-related macular degeneration. *Arch Ophthalmol* 2001;119:1191-1199.

9. Ouchi, M., et al. A novel relation of fatty acid with age-related macular degeneration. *Ophthalmologica* 2002;216:363-367.

10. Sheddon, JM, et al. Progression of age-related macular degeneration: association with dietary fat, transunsaturated fat, nuts, and fish intake. *Arch Ophthalmol* 2003;121:1728-1737.

11. Bhuyan, KC and Bhuyan, DK. Lipid peroxidation in cataract of the human. *Life Sci* 1986;38:1463-1471.

12. Wu, Y, et al. Oxidative stress: implications for the development of diabetic retinopathy and antioxidant therapeutic perspectives. *Oxid Med Cell Longev* 2014:752387.

13. Chang, CK and LoCicero, J III. Overexpressed nuclear factor kB correlates with enhanced expression of interleukin-1β and inducible nitric oxide synthase in aged murine lungs to endotoxic stress. *Annals of Thoracic Surgery* 2004;77:1222-1227.

14. Tewfik, IH, et al. The effect of intermittent heating on some chemical parameters of refined oils used in Egypt. A public health nutrition concern. *Int J Food Sci Nutr* 1998;49:339-342.

15. Jurgens, G, et al. Immunostaining of human autopsy aortas with antibodies to modified apolipoprotein B and apoprotein(a). *Arterioscler Thromb* 1993;13:1689-1699.

16. Srivastava, S, et al. Identification of cardiac oxidoreductase(s) involved in the metabolism of the lipid peroxidation-derived aldehyde-4-hydroxynonenal. *Biochem J* 1998;329:469-475.

17. Nakamura, K, et al. Carvedilol decreases elevated oxidative stress in human failing myocardium. *Circulation* 2002;105:2867-2871.

18. Pratico, D and Delanty, N. Oxidative injury in diseases of the central nervous system: focus on Alzheimer's disease. *American Journal of Medicine* 2000;109:577-585.

19. Markesbery, WR and Carney, JM. Oxidative alterations in Alzheimer's disease. *Brain Pathology* 1999;9;133-146.

20. Kritchevsky, D and Tepper, SA. Cholesterol vehicle in experimental atherosclerosis. 9. Comparison of heated corn oil and heated olive oil. *J Atheroscler Res* 1967;7:647-651.

21. Seddon, JM, et al. Progression of age-related macular degeneration: association with dietary fat, transunsaturated fat, nuts, and fish intake. *Arch Ophthalmol* 2003;121(12):1728-1737.

22. Ouchi, M, et al. A novel relation of fatty acid with age-related macular degeneration. *Ophthalmologica* 2002;216(5):363-367.

23. Seddon, JM, et al. Dietary fat and risk for advanced age-related macular degeneration. *Arch Ophthalmol* 2001;119(8):1191-1199.

24. Raloff, J. 1996. Unusual fats lose heart-friendly image. *Science News* 1996;150:87.

25. Mensink, RP and Katan, MB. 1990. Effect of dietary trans fatty acids on high-density and low-density lipoprotein cholesterol levels in healthy subjects. *N Eng J Med* 323(7):439-445.

26. Willett, WC, et al. 1993. Intake of trans fatty acids and risk of coronary heart disease among women. *Lancet* 341(8845):581-585.

27. Booyens, J and Louwrens, CC. The Eskimo diet. Prophylactic effects ascribed to the balanced presence of natural cis unsaturated fatty acids and

to the absence of unnatural trans and cis isomers of unsaturated fatty acids. *Med Hypoth* 1986;21:387-408

28. Grandgirard, A, et al. Incorporation of trans long-chain n-3 polyunsaturated fatty acids in rat brain structures and retina. *Lipids* 1994;29:251-258.

29. Pamplona, R, et al. Low fatty acid unsaturation: a mechanism for lowered lipoperoxidative modification of tissue proteins in mammalian species with long life spans. *J Gerontol A Biol Sci Med Sci* 2000;55:B286-B291.

30. Cha, YS and Sachan, DS. Opposite effects of dietary saturated and unsaturated fatty acids on ethanol-pharmacokinetics, triglycerides and carnitines. *J Am Coll Nutr* 1994;13:338-343.

31. Siri-Tarino, PW, et al. Meta-analysis of prospective cohort studies evaluating the association of saturated fat with cardiovascular disease. *Am J Clin Nutr* 2010;91:535-546.

32. Ramsden, CE, et al. Use of dietary linoleic acid for secondary prevention of coronary heart disease and death: evaluation of recovered data for the Sydney Diet Heart Study and updated meta-analysis. *BMJ* 2013 Feb 4;346:e8707. doi:10.1136/bmj.e8707.

33. Calder, PC. Old study sheds new light on the fatty acids and cardiovascular health debate. *BMJ* 2013 Feb 4;346:f493. doi:10.1136/bmj.f493.

34. Chowdhury, R, et al. Association of dietary, circulating, and supplement fatty acids with coronary risk: a systematic review and meta-analysis. *Ann Intern Med* 2014;160:398-406.

Chapter 7: Top Nutrients for Good Eye Health

1. van Lieshout, M, et al. Bioefficacy of beta-carotene dissolved in oil studied in children in Indonesia. *Am J Clin Nutr* 2001;73:949-958.

2. Sauberlich, HE, et al. Vitamin A metabolism and requirements in the human studied with the use of labeled retinol. *Vitam Horm* 1974;32:251-275.

3. http://ods.od.nih.gov/factsheets/VitaminA-HealthProfessional/

4. Usoro, OB and Mousa, SA. Vitamin E forms in Alzheimer's disease: a review of controversial and clinical experiences. *Crit Rev Food Sci Nutr* 2010;50:414-419.

5. A Randomized, placebo-controlled, clinical trial of high-dose supplementation with vitamins C and E and beta carotene for age-related cataract and vision loss. *Arch Ophthalmol* 2001;119:1439-1452.

6. Teikari, J, et al. Long-term supplementation with alpha-tocopherol and beta-carotene and age-related cataract. *Acta Ophthalmol Scand* 1997;75:634-640.

7. Sperduto, RD, et al. The Linxian Catract Studies: two nutritional intervention trails. *Arch Ophthalmol* 1993;111:1246-1253.

8. Snodderly, DM. Evidence for protection against age-related macular

degeneration by carotenoids and antioxidant vitamins. *Am J Clin Nutr* 1995;62(Suppl):1448S-1461S.

9. Seddon, JM, et al. Dietary carotenoids, vitamins A, C, and E and advanced age-related macular degeneration. Eye disease case-control study group. *JAMA* 1994;272:1413-1420.

10. Nagai, N, et al. Suppression of diabetic-induced retinal inflammation by blocking the angiotensin II type 1 receptor or it downstream nuclear factor-kappaB pathway. *Invest Ophthalmol Vis Sci* 2007;48:4342-4350.

11. Chasan-Taber, L, et al. A prospective study of carotenoids and vitamin A intakes and risk of cataract extraction in US women. *Am J Clin Nutr* 1999;70:509-516.

12. Sommerburg, O, et al. Fruits and vegetables that are sources for lutein and zeaxanthin: the macular pigment in human eyes. *Br J Ophthalmol* 1998;82:907-910.

13. Chong, EW, et al. Dietary omega-3 fatty acid and fish intake in the primary prevention of age-related macular degeneration: a systemic review and meta-analysis. *Arch Ophthalmol* 2008;126:826-833.

14. Hammes, HP, et al. Acceleration of experimental diabetic retinopathy in the rat by omega-3 fatty acids. *Diabetologia* 1996;39:251-255.

15. Bourre, JM. Free radicals, polyunsaturated fatty acids, cell death, brain aging. *CR Seances Soc Biol Fil* 1988;182:5-36.

16. Esterhuyse, AJ, et al. Dietary red palm oil supplementation protects against the consequences of global ischemia in the isolated perfused rat heart. *Asia Pac J Clin Nutr* 2005;14:340-347.

17. Khanna, S, et al. Molecular basis of vitamin E action: tocotrienol modulates 12-lipoxygenase, a key moderator of glutamate-induced neurodegeneration. *J Biol Chem* 2003;278:43508-43515.

18. Holmberg, S, et al. Food choices and coronary heart disease: a population based cohort study of rural Swedish men with 12 years of follow-up. *Int J Environ Res Public Health* 2009;6:2626-2638.

19. Conlon, LE, et al. Coconut oil enhances tomato carotenoid tissue accumulation compared to safflower oil in the Mongolian gerbil (Meriones unguiculatus). *J Agric Food Chem* 2012;60:8386-8394.

20. Nidhi, B, et al. Dietary fatty acid determines the intestinal absorption of lutein in lutein deficient mice. *Foods Research International* 2014;64:256-263.

21. Gleize, B, et al. Effect of type of TAG fatty acids on lutein and zeaxanthin bioavailability. *Br J Nutr* 2013;110:1-10.

22. Hayatullina, Z, et al. Virgin coconut oil supplementation prevents bone loss in osteoporosis rat model. *Evid Based Complement Alternat Med* 2012 1012:237236.

23. Wang, X, et al. Enteral nutrition improves clinical outcome and shortens hospital stay after cancer surgery. *J Invest Surg* 2010;23:309-313.

24. Nomura, Y, et al. Importance of nutritional status in recovery from acute cholecystitis: benefit from enteral nutrition supplementation including medium chain triglycerides. *Nihon Shokakibyo Gakkai Zasshi* 2007;104:1352-1358.

25. Meydani, SN, et al. Effect of age and dietary fat (fish, corn and coconut oils) on tocopherol status of C57BL/6Nia mice. *Lipids* 1987;22:345-350.

26. Arunima, S and Rajamohan, T. Effect of virgin coconut oil enriched diet on the antioxidant status and paraoxonase 1 activity in ameliorating the oxidative stress in rats – a comparative study. *Food Funct* 2013;4:1402-1409.

27. Goodrow, EF, et al. Consumption of one egg per day increases serum lutein and zeaxanthin concentrations in older adults without altering serum lipid and lipoprotein cholesterol concentrations. *J Nutr* 2006;136:2519-2524.

28. Wenzel, AJ, et al. A 12-week egg intervention increases serum zeaxanthin and macular pigment optical density in women. *J Nutr* 2006;126:2568-2573.

Chapter 8: The Miracle of Ketones

1. Walford, RL. Calorie restriction: eat less, eat better, live longer. *Life Extension* 1998;Feb:19-22.

2. Bruce-Keller, AJ, et al. Food restriction reduces brain damage and improves behavioral outcome following excitotoxic and metabolic insults. *Ann Neurol* 1999;45:8-15.

3. Dubey, A, et al. Effect of age and caloric intake on protein oxidation in different brain regions and on behavioral functions of the mouse. *Arch Biochem Biophys* 1996;333:189-197.

4. Duan, W and Mattson, MP. Dietary restriction and 2-deoxyglucose administration improve behavioral outcome and reduce degeneration of dopaminergic neurons in models of Parkinson's disease. *J Neurosci Res* 1999;57:195-206.

5. Mattson, MP. Neuroprotective signaling and the aging brain: take away my food and let me run. *Brain Res* 2000;886:47-53.

6. Matthews, AG. The lens and cataracts. Vet Clin North Am Equine Pract 2004;20:393-415.

7. Robman, I and Taylor, H. External factors in the development of cataract. *Eye* 2005;19:1074-1082.

8.Taylor, A., et al. Moderate caloric restriction delays cataract formation in the Emory mouse. *Faseb J* 1989;3:1741-1746.

9. Obin, M, et al. Calorie restriction modulates age-dependent changes in the retinas of Brown Norway rats. *Mech Ageing Dev* 2000;114:133-147.

10. LI, D, et al. Caloric restriction retards age-related changes in rat retina. *Biochem Biophys Res Commun* 2003;309:457-463.

11. Katz, ML, et al. Dietary restriction slows age pigment accumulation in the retinal pigment epithelium. *Invest Ophthalmol Vis Sci* 1993;34:3297-3302.

12. Li, U and Wolf NS. Effects of age and long-term caloric restriction on the aqueous collecting channel in the mouse eye. *J Glaucoma* 1997;6:18-22.

13. Kawai, SI, et al. Modeling of risk factors for the degeneration of retinal ganglion cells after ischemia/reperfusion in rats: effects of age, caloric restriction, diabetes, pigmentation, and glaucoma. *Faseb J* 2001;15:1285-12887.

14. Kim, KY, et al. Neuronal susceptibility to damage: comparison of the retinas of young, old and old/caloric restricted rats before and after transient ischemia. *Neurobiol Aging* 2004;25:491-500.

15. Mattson, MP. Neuroprotective signaling and the aging brain: take away my food and let me run. *Brain res* 2000;886:47-53.

16. Colcombe, SJ, et al. Aerobic exercise training increases brain volume in aging humans. *J Gerontol A Biol Sci Med Sci* 2006;61:1166-1170.

17. Larson, EB, et al. Exercise is associated with reduced risk for incident dementia among persons 65 years of age or older. *Ann Intern Med* 2006;144:73-81.

18. Lautenschlager, NT, et al. Effect of physical activity on cognitive function in older adults at risk for Alzheimer disease: a randomized trial. *JAMA* 2008;300:1027-1037.

19. Honea, RA, et al. Cardiorespiratory fitness and preserved medial temporal lobe volume in Alzheimer disease. *Alzheimer Dis Assoc Disord* 2009;23:188-197.

20. Faherty, CJ, et al. Environmental enrichment in adulthood eliminates neuronal death in experimental Parkinsonism. *Brain Res Mol Brain Res* 2005;134:170-179.

21. Williams, PT. Prospective study of incident age-related macular degeneration in relation to vigorous physical activity during a 7-year follow-up. *Invest Ophthalmol Vis Sci* 2009;50:101-106.

22. Lawson, EC, et al. Aerobic exercise protects retinal function and structure form light-induced retinal degeneration. *Journal of Neuroscience* 2014;34:2406-2412.

23. Rojas Vega, S. et al. Effect of resistance exercise on serum levels of growth factors in humans. *Horm Metab Res* 2010;42:982-986.

24. Goekint, M, et al Strength training does not influence serum brain-derived neurotrophic factor. *Eur J Appl Phsiol* 2010;110:285-293.

25. Knaepen, K, et al. Neuroplasticity—exercise-induced response of peripheral brain-derived neurotrophic factor: a systemic review of

experimental studies in human subjects. *Sports Med* 2010;40:765-801.

26. Coelho, FG, et al. Physical exercise modulates peripheral levels of brain-derived neurotrophic factor (BDNF): a systematic review of experimental studies in the elderly. *Arch Gerontol Geriatr* 2013;56:10-15.

27. Williams, PT. Prospective study of incident age-related macular degeneration in relation to vigorous physical activity during a 7-year follow-up. *Invest Ophthalmol Vis Sci* 2009;50:101-106.

28. Nordli, DR Jr, et al. Experience with the ketogenic diet in infants. *Pediatrics* 2001;108:129-133.

29. Pulsifer, MB, et al. Effects of ketogenic diet on development and behavior: preliminary report of a prospective study. *Dev Med Child Neurol* 2001;43:301-306.

30. Husain, AM, et al. Diet therapy for narcolepsy. *Nuerology* 2004;62:2300-2302.

31. Evangeliou, A, et al. Application of a ketogenic diet in children with autistic behavior: pilot study. *J Child Neurol* 2003;18:113-118.

32. Strahlman, RS. Can ketosis help migraine sufferers? A case report. Headache 2006;46:182.

33. Murphy, P, et al. The antidepressant properties of the ketogenic diet. *Biological Psychiatry* 2004;56:981-983.

34. Gasior, M, et al. Neuroprotective and disease-modifying effects of the ketogenic diet. *Behav Pharmacol* 2006;17:431-439.

35. Van der Auwera, I, et al. A ketogenic diet reduces amyloid beta 40 and 42 in mouse model of Alzheimer's disease. *Nutrition* 2005;2:28.

36. Zhao, Z, et al. A ketogenic diet as a potential novel therapeutic intervention in amyotrophic lateral sclerosis. *BMC Neuroscience* 2006;7:29.

37. Duan, W, et al. Dietary restriction normalizes glucose metabolism and BDNF levels, slows disease progression, and increases survival in huntingtin mutant mice. *Proc Natl Acad Sci USA* 2003;100:2911-2916.

38. Kashiwaya, Y, et al. D-beta-hydroxybutyrate protects neurons in models of Alzheimer's and Parkinson's disease. *Proc Natl Acad Sci USA* 2000;97:5440-5444.

39. Tieu, K, et al. D-beta-hydroxybutyrate rescues mitochondrial respiration and mitigates features of Parkinson disease. *J Clin Invest* 2003;112:892-901.

40. VanItallie, TB, et al. Treatment of Parkinson disease with diet-induced hyperketonemia: a feasibility study. *Neurology* 2005;64:728-730.

41. Van der Auwera, I, et al. A ketogenic diet reduces amyloid beta 40 and 42 in a mouse model of Alzheimer's disease. *Nutr Metab (London)* 2005;2:28.

42. Studzinski, CM, et al. Induction of ketosis may improve mitochondrial function and decrease steady-state amyloid-beta precursor protein (AAPP) levels in the aged dog. *Brain Res* 2008;1226:209-217.

43. Costantini, LC, et al. Hypometabolism as a therapeutic target in Alzheimer's disease. *BMC Neuroscience* 2008;9:S16.

44. Suzuki, M, et al. Beta-hydroxybutyrate, a cerebral function improving agent, protects rat brain against ischemic damage caused by permanent and transient focal cerebral ischemia. *Jpn J Phamacol* 2002;89:36-43.

45. Suzuki, M, et al. Effect of beta-hydroxybutyrate, a cerebral function improving agent, on cerebral hypoxia, anoxia and ischemia in mice and rats. *Jpn J Phamacol* 2001;87:143-150.

46. Imamura, K, et al. D-beta-hydroxybutyrate protects dopaminergic SH-SY5Y cells in a rotenone model of Parkinson's disease. *J Neuroscie Res* 2006;84:1376-1384.

47. Maalouf, M, et al. The neuroprotective properties of calorie restriction, the ketogenic diet, and ketone bodies. *Brain Res Rev* 2009; 59:293-315.

48. Zarnowski, T, et al. A ketogenic diet may offer neuroprotection in glaucoma and mitochondrial diseases of the optic nerve. *MEHDI Ophthalmology Journal* 2012;1:45-49.

49. Robinson, AM and Williamson, DH. Physiological roles of ketone bodies as substrates and signals in mammalian tissues. *Physiol Rev* 1980;60:143-187.

50. Rosedale, R, et al. Clinical experience of a diet designed to reduce aging. J Appl Res 2009;9:159-165.

51. Gaziano, JM, et al. Fasting triglycerides, high-density lipoprotein, and risk of myocardial infarction. *Circulation* 1997;96:2520-2525.

52. Accurso, A, et al. Dietary carbohydrate restriction in type 2 diabetes mellitus and metabolic syndrome: time for a critical appraisal. *Nutrition & Metabolism* 2008;5:9.

53. Neilsen, JV and Joensson, EA. Low-carbohydrate diet in type 2 diabetes: stable improvement of bodyweight and glycemic control during 44 months follow-up. *Nutrition & Metabolism* 2008;5:14.

54. Volek, JS and Feinman, RD. Carbohydrate restriction improves the features of metabolic syndrome. Metabolic syndrome may be defined by the response to carbohydrate restriction. *Nutrition & Metabolism* 2005;2:31.

55. Forsythe, CE, et al. Comparison of low fat and low carbohydrate diets on circulating fatty acid composition and markers of inflammation. *Lipids* 2008;43:65-77.

56. Volek, JS, et al. Modification of lipoproteins by very low-carbohydrate diets. *J Nutr* 2005;135:1339-1342.

57. Craft, S and Watson, GS. Insulin and neurodegenerative disease: shared and specific mechanisms. *Lancet Neurology* 2004;3:169-178.

58. Martin, PM, et al. Expression of the sodium-coupled monocarbonxylate transporters SMCT1 (SLC5A8) and SMCT2 (SLCA12) in retina. *Invest Ophthalmol Vis Sci* 2007;48:3356-3363.

59. Suzuki, M, et al. Effect of beta-hydroxybutyrate, a cerebral function improving agent, on cerebral hypoxia, anoxia, and ischemia in mice and rates. *Jpn J Pharmacol* 2001;87:143-150.

60. Smith, SL, et al. KTX 0101:A Potential metabolic approach to cytoprotection in major surgery and neurological disorders. *CNS Drug Rev* 2005;11:113-140.

61. Veech, RL. The therapeutic implications of ketone bodies: the effects of ketone bodies in pathological conditions: ketosis, ketogenic diet, redox states, insulin resistance, and mitochondrial metabolism. *Prostaglandins, Leukotrienes and Essential Fatty Acids* 2004;70:309-319.

62. Maalouf, M, et al. The neuroprotective properties of calorie restriction, the ketogenic diet, and ketone bodies. *Brain Res Rev* 2009;59:293-315.

63. Pedersen, BK, et al. Role of exercise-induced brain-derived neurotrophic factor production in the regulation of energy homeostasis in mammals. *Exp Physiol* 2009;94:1153-1160.

64. Krabble, KS, et al. Brain-derived neurotrophic factor (BDNF) and type 2 diabetes. *Diabetologia* 2007;50:431-438.

65. Schiffer, T, et al. Effects of strength and endurance training on brain-derived neurotrophic factor and insulin-like growth factor 1 in humans. *Horm Metab Res* 2009;41:250-254.

66. Krabbe, KS, et al. Brain-derived neurotrophic factor (BDNF) and type 2 diabetes. *Diabetologia* 2007;50:431-438.

67. Maalouf, M, et al. Ketones inhibit mitochondrial production of reactive oxygen species production following glutamate excitotoxicity by increasing NADH oxidation. *Neuroscience* 2007;145:256-264.

68. Koper, JW, et al. Acetoacetate and glucose as substrates for lipid synthesis for rat brain oligodendrocytes and astrocytes in serum-free culture. *Biochim Biophys Acta* 1984;796:20-26.

69. Yeh, YY, et al. Ketone bodies serve as important precursors of brain lipid in the developing rat. *Lipids* 1977;12:957-964.

70. Wu, PY, et al. Medium-chain triglycerides in infant formulas and their relation to plasma ketone body concentrations. *Pediatr Res* 1986;20:338-341.

71. Fischer, D. Stimulating axonal regeneration of mature retinal ganglion cells and overcoming inhibitory signaling. Cell Tissue Res 2012;349:79-85.

72. Mansour-Robaey, S, et al. Effects of ocular injury and administration of brain-derived neurotrophic factor on survival and regrowth of axontomized retinal ganglion cells. *Proc Natl Acad Sci* 1994;91:1632-1636.

73. Thaler, S, et al. Neuroprotection by acetoacetate and beta-hydroxybutyrate against NMDA-induced RGC damage in rat-possible involvement of kynurenic acid. *Graefes Arch Clin Exp Ophthalmo* 2010;248:1729-1735.

74. Weibel, D, et al. Brain-derived neurotrophic factor (BDNF) prevents lesion-induced axonal die-back in young rat optic nerve. *Brain Res* 1995;679:249-254.

75. Okoye, G, et al. Increased expression of brain-derived neurotrophic factor preserves retinal function and slows cell death from rhodopsin mutation or oxidative damage. *Journal of Neuroscience* 2003;23:4164-4172.

Chapter 9: Coconut Ketones

1. Bergen, SS Jr., et al. Hyperketonemia induced in man by medium-chain triglyceride. *Diabetes* 1966;15:723-725.

2. http://coconutresearchcenter.org/60_persons_with_dimentia_study.htm

3. Wlaz, P, et al. Anticonvulsant profile of caprylic acid, a main constituent of the medium-chain triglyceride (MCT) ketogenic diet, in mice. *Neuropharmacology* 2012;62:1882-1889.

4. Sills, MA, et al. The Medium chain triglyceride diet and intractable epilepsy. *Arch Dis Child* 1986;61:1168-1172.

5. Huttenlocher, PR, et al. Medium-chain triglycerides as a therapy for intractable childhood epilepsy. *Neurology* 1971;21:1097-1103.

6. Pan, Y, et al. Dietary supplementation with medium-chain TAG has long-lasting cognition-enhancing effects in aged dogs. *Br J Nutr* 2010;103:1746-1754.

7. Reger MA, et al. Effects of beta-hydroxybutyrate on cognition in memory-impaired adults. *Neurobiol Aging* 2004;25:311-314.

8. Nafar, F and Mearow, KM. Coconut oil attenuates the effects of amyloid-beta on cortical neurons in vitro. *J Alzheimers Dis* 2014;39:233-7.

9. Zhao, W, et al. Caprylic triglyceride as a novel therapeutic approach to effectively improve the performance and attenuate the symptoms due to the motor neuron loss in ALS disease. *PLoS One* 2012. DOI:10.1371/journal. pone.0049191.

10. Twyman, D. Nutritional management of the critically ill neurologic patient. *Crit Care Clin* 1997;13:39-49.

11. Calon, B, et al. Long-chain versus medium and long-chain triglyceride-based fat emulsion in parental nutrition of severe head trauma patients. *Infusionstherapie* 1990;17:246-248.

12. Katz, B and Rimmer, S. Ophthalmic manifestations of Alzheimer's disease. *Surv Ophthalmol* 1989;104:113-120.

13. Berisha, F, et al. Retinal Abnormalities in Early Alzheimer's Disease. *Invest Ophthalmol Vis Sci* 2007;48:2285-2289.

14. Iseri, PK, et al. Relationship between cognitive impairment and retinal morphological and visual functional abnormalities in Alzheimer disease. *J Neuroophthalmol* 2006;26:18-24.

Chapter 10: Coconut Therapy

1. Chiu, CJ, et al. Dietary carbohydrate and the progression of age-related macular degeneration: a prospective study form the Age-Related Eye Disease Study. *Am J Clin Nutr* 2007;86:1210-1218.

2. Chiu, CJ, et al. Dietary glycemic index and carbohydrate in relation to early age-related macular degeneration. *Am J Clin Nutr* 2006;83:880-886.

3. Chiu, CJ, et al. Carbohydrate intake and glycemic index in relation to the odds of early cortical and nuclear lens opacities. *Am J Clin Nutr* 2005;81:1411-1416.

4. Stitt, AW. The maillard reaction in eye diseases. *Ann NY Acad Sci* 20005;1043:582-597.

5. Chiu, CJ, et al. Association between dietary glycemic index and age-related macular degeneration in nondiabetic participants in the Age-Related Eye Disease Study. *Am J Clin Nutr* 2007;86:180-188.

6. Kamuren, ZT, et al. Effects of low-carbohydrate diet and Pycnogenol treatment on retinal antioxidant enzymes in normal and diabetic rats. *J Ocul Pharmacol Ther* 2006;22:10-18.

7. Turner, N, et al. Enhancement of muscle mitochondrial oxidative capacity and alterations in insulin action are lipid species dependent: potent tissue-specific effects of medium chain fatty acids. *Diabetes* 2009;58:2547-2554.

8. Poplawski, MM, et al. Reversal of diabetic nephropathy by a ketogenic diet. *PLoS One* 2011;6:e18604.

9. Ola, MS, et al. Reduced levels of brain derived neurotrophic factor (BDNF) in the serum of diabetic retinopathy patients and in the retina of diabetic rats. *Cell Mol Neurobiol* 2013;33:359-367.

10. Zarnowski, T and Kosior-Jarecka, E. Progression of normal tension glaucoma in Kearns-Sayre syndrome over 10 years. *Clin Experiment Ophthalmol* 2012;40:218-220.

11. Chang, EE and Goldberg, JL. Glaucoma 2.0: neuroprotection, neuroregeneration, neuroenhancement.. *Ophthalmology* 2012;119:979-986.

12. Bayer, AU, et al. High occurrence rate of glaucoma among patients with Alzheimer's disease. *Eur Neurol.* 2002;47(3):165-168.

13. Tamura H, et al. High frequency of open-angle glaucoma in Japanese patients with Alzheimer's disease. *J Neurol Sci* 2006;246(1-2):79-83.

14. Helmer C, et al. Is there a link between open-angle glaucoma and dementia?: The Three-City—Alienor Cohort. *Ann Neurol* 2013;74:171-179

15. Ko, ML, et al. Patterns of retinal ganglion cell survival after brain-derived neurotrophic factor administration in hypertensive eyes of rats. *Neurosci Lett* 2001:305:139-142.

16. Gopikrishna, V, et al. A quantitative analysis of coconut water: a new storage media for avulsed teeth. *Oral Surg Oral Med Oral Pathol Oral Radiol Endod* 2008;105:e61-65.

17. Silva, JR, et al. Effect of coconut water and Braun-Collins solutions at different temperatures and incubation times on the morphology of goat preantral follicles preserved in vitro. *Theriogenology* 2000;54:809-822.

18. Gopikrishna, V, et al. Comparison of coconut water, propolis, HBSS, and milk on PDL cell survival. *J Endod* 2008;34:587-589.

19. Rattan, SIS and Clark, BFC. Kinetin delays the onset of ageing characteristics in human fibroblasts. *Biochem Biophys Res* 1994;201:665-672.

20. Kowalska, E. Influence of kinetin (6-furfurylo-amino-purine) on human fibroblasts in the cell culture. *Folia Morphol* 1992;51:109-118.

21. Radenahmad, N, et al. Young coconut juice, a potential therapeutic agent that could significantly reduce some pathologies associated with Alzheimer's disease: novel findings. *Br J Nutr* 2011;105:738-746.

22. Choi, SJ, et al. Zeatin prevents amyloid beta-induced neurotoxicity and scopolamine-induced cognitive deficits. *J Med Food* 2009;12:271-277.

23. Vicanova, J, et al. Epidermal and dermal characteristics in skin equivalent after systemic and topical application of skin care ingredients. *Ann N Y Acad Sci* 2006;1067:337-342.

24. Kimura, T and Doi, K. Depigmentation and rejuvenation effects of kinetin on the aged skin of hairless descendants of Mexican hairless dogs. *Rejuvenation Res* 2004;7:32-39.

25. Hipkiss, AR. On the "struggle between chemistry and biology during aging"—implications for DNA repair, apoptosis and proteolysis, and a novel route of intervention. *Biogerontology* 20012:173-178.

26. Mantena, SK, et al. In vitro evaluation of antioxidant properties of Cocos nucifera Linn. Water. *Nahrung* 2003;47:126-131.

27. Loki, AL and Rajamohan, T. Hepatoprotective and antioxidant effect of tender coconut water on carbon tetrachloride induced liver injury in rats. *Indian J Biochem Biophys* 2003;40:354-357.

28. da Fonseca, A, et al. Constituents and antioxidant activity of two varieties of coconut water (Cocos nucifera L.). *Rev Bras Farmacogn* 2009;19 (1b).

29. Sharma, SP, et al Plant-growth hormone kinetin delays aging, prolongs the life-span and slows down development of the fruitfly Zaprionus paravittiger. *Biochem Biophys Res Comm* 1995;216:1067-1071.

30. Du, Q, et al. Study on tissue culture and plant regeneration of Nervilia fordii. *Zhongguo Zhong Yao Za Zhi* 2005;30:812-814.

31. Souza, BD, et al. Viability of human periodontal ligament fibroblasts in milk, Hank's balanced salt solution and coconut water as storage media. *Int Endod J* 2011;44:111-115.

32. Silva, MA, et al. Recovery and cryopreservation of epididymal sperm from agouti (Dasiprocta aguti) using powdered coconut water (ACP-109c) and Tris extenders. *Theriogenology* 2011;76:1084-1089.

33. Lima, GL, et al. Short-term storage of canine preantral ovarian follicles using a powdered coconut water-based medium. *Theriogenology* 2010;74:146-152.

34. Silva, AE, et al. The influence of powdered coconut water (ACP-318) in in vitro maturation of canine oocytes. *Reprod Domest Anim* 2010;45:1042-1046.

35. Babizhayev, MA. Biomarkers and special features of oxidative stress in the anterior segment of the eye linked to lens cataract and the trabecular meshwork injury in primary open-angle glaucoma: challenges of dual combination therapy with N-acetylcarnosine lubricant eye drops and oral formulation of nonhydrolyzed carnosine. *Fundam Clin Pharmacol* 2012;26:86-117.

36. Farooq, M, et al. GluA2 AMPA glutamate receptor subunit exhibits condon 607 Q/R RNA editing in the lens. *Biochemical and Biophysical Research Communications* 2012;418:273-277.

37. Miljanovi B, et al. Relation between dietary n-3 and n-6 fatty acids and clinically diagnosed dry eye syndrome in women. *Am J Clin Nutr* 2005;82:887–893.

38. Intahphuak, S, et al. Anti-inflammatory, analgesic, and antipyretic activities of virgin coconut oil. *Pharm Biol* 2010;48:151-157.

39. http://www.google.com/patents/US20040197340, accessed 1/1/2014.

40. http://www.google.com.ar/patents/US20110152307, accessed 1/1/2014.

41. Dayrit, CS. *The Truth About Coconut Oil: The Drugstore in A Bottle.* Anvil Publishing, Inc., Pasig City, Philippines, 2005.

42. http://news.utoronto.ca/understanding-gwyneth-paltrows-oil-pulling-regime.

43. Chandrasekar, B, et al. Effects of calorie restriction on transforming growth factor beta 1 and proinflammatory cytokines in murine Sjogren's syndrome. *Clin Immunol Immunopathol* 1995;76(3 Pt 1):291-296.

Chapter 11: The Low-Carbohydrate Diet

1. Brighenti, F, et al. Effect of neutralized and native vinegar on blood glucose and acetate responses to a mixed meal in healthy subjects. *Eur J Clin Nutr* 1995;49:242-247.

2. Johnston, CS, et al. Vinegar improves insulin sensitivity to a high-carbohydrate meal in subjects with insulin resistance or type 2 diabetes. *Diabetes Care* 2004;27:281-282.

Index

The Coconut Ketogenic Diet:
Supercharge Your Metabolism, Revitalize Thyroid Function, and Lose Excess Weight

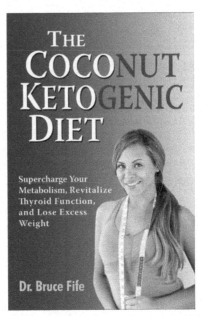

You can enjoy eating rich, full-fat foods and lose weight without counting calories or suffering from hunger. The secret is a high-fat, ketogenic diet. Our bodies need fat. It's necessary for optimal health. It's also necessary in order to lose weight safely and naturally.

Low-fat diets have been heavily promoted for the past three decades, and as a result we are fatter now than ever before. Obviously, there is something wrong with the low-fat approach to weight loss. This book exposes many common myths and misconceptions about fats and weight loss and explains why low-fat diets don't work. It also reveals new, cutting-edge research on one of the world's most exciting weight loss aids—coconut oil—and how you can use it to power up your metabolism, boost your energy, improve thyroid function, and lose unwanted weight.

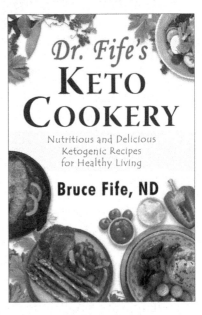

This revolutionary weight loss program is designed to keep you both slim and healthy using wholesome, natural foods, and the most health-promoting fats. It has proven successful in helping those suffering from obesity, diabetes, heart and circulatory problems, low thyroid function, chronic fatigue, high blood pressure, high cholesterol, and many other conditions.

Dr. Fife's Keto Cookery
Nutritious and Delicious Ketogenic Recipes for Healthy Living

What do you eat on a ketogenic diet? No need to worry, Dr. Fife has written a easy-to-follow cookbook filled with his all-time favorite ketogenic recipes. The majority of the recipes are quick and easy, designed for everyday use for busy people. This is an invaluable resource for anyone thinking of going keto.

Coconut Water for Health and Healing

Coconut water is a refreshing beverage that is a powerhouse of nutrition containing a complex blend of vitamins, minerals, amino acids, antioxidants, enzymes, health enhancing growth hormones, and other phytonutrients.

Because its electrolyte (ionic min-eral) content is similar to human plasma, it has gained international acclaim as a natural sports drink for oral rehydration. As such, it has proven superior to commercial sports drinks.

Coconut water's unique nutritional profile gives it the power to balance body chemistry, ward off disease, fight cancer, and retard aging. History and folklore credit coconut water with remarkable healing powers, which medical science is now confirming.

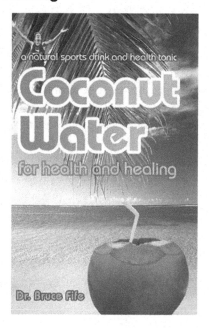

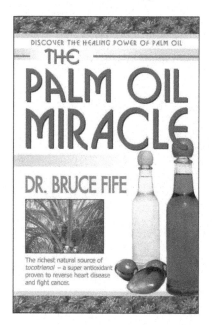

The Palm Oil Miracle

Palm oil has been used as both a food and a medicine for thousands of years. it was prized by the pharaohs of ancient Egypt as a sacred food. In tropical Africa and Southeast Asia it is an integral part of a healthy diet.

Palm oil possesses excellent cooking properties. It is more heat stable than other vegetable oils and imparts in foods and baked goods superior taste, texture, and quality.

Palm oil is one of the world's healthiest oils. It is currently being used by doctors and government agencies to treat specific illnesses and improve nutritional status. Recent medical studies have shown that palm oil, particularly virgin (red) palm oil, can protect against many common health problems.

STOP ALZHEIMER'S NOW!

How to Prevent and Reverse Dementia, Parkinson's, ALS, Multiple Sclerosis, and Other Neurodegenerative Disorders

By Bruce Fife, ND. Foreword by Russell L. Blaylock, MD

More than 35 million people have dementia today. Alzheimer's disease is the most common form of dementia. The number of people affected continues to increase every year.

Alzheimer's *not* a part of the normal aging process. While aging is a risk factor for neurodegeneration, it is not the cause. Alzheimer's can be prevented and successfully treated.

This book outlines a program using ketone therapy and diet that is backed by decades of medical and clinical research and has proven successful in restoring mental function and improving both brain and overall health. You will learn how to prevent and even reverse symptoms associated with Alzheimer's disease, Parkinson's disease, amyotrophic lateral sclerosis (ALS), multiple sclerosis (MS), Huntington's disease, epilepsy, diabetes, stroke, and various forms of dementia.

The information in this book is useful not only for those who are suffering from neurodegenerative disease but for anyone who wants to be spared from ever encountering one or more of these devastating afflictions. These diseases don't just happen overnight. They take years, often decades, to develop. In the case of Alzheimer's disease, approximately 70 percent the brain cells responsible for memory are destroyed *before* symptoms become noticeable.

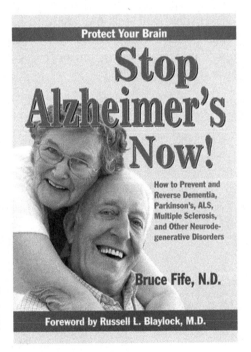

You *can* stop Alzheimer's and other neurodegenerative diseases before they take over your life. The best time to start is now.

Visit Us on the Web

P⒝ Piccadilly Books, Ltd.

www.piccadillybooks.com

Made in USA - Kendallville, IN
1239272_9780941599962
02.25.2021 0812